NAIL
ART
PROJECTS

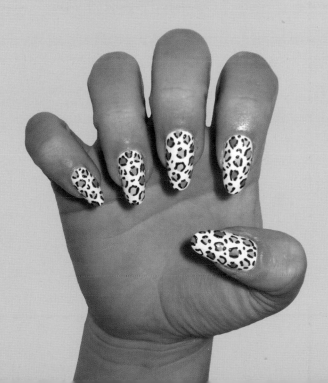

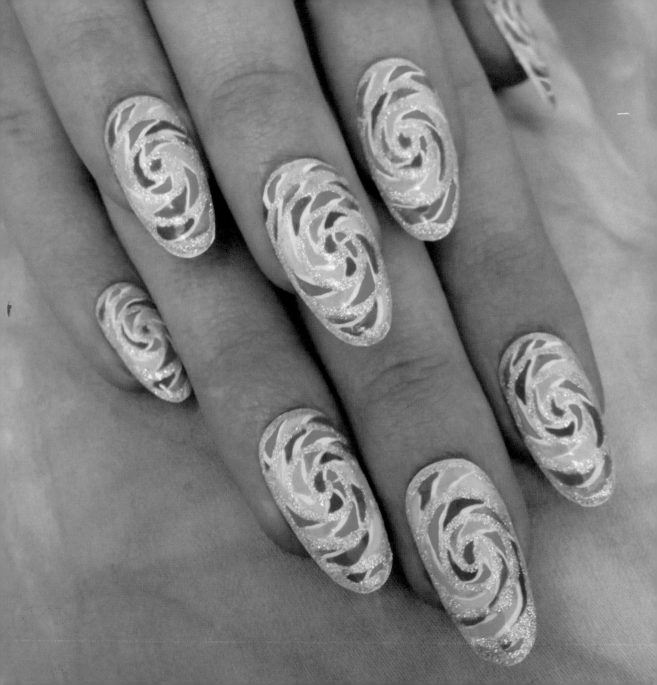

NAIL ART PROJECTS

Eye-catching and stylish designs by salon professionals

HELENA BIGGS

ARCTURUS

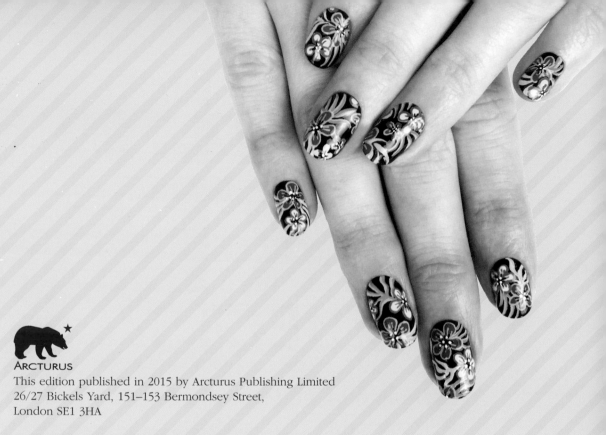

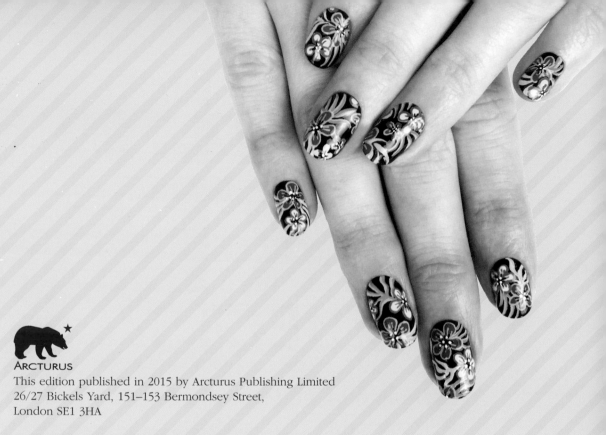

ARCTURUS

This edition published in 2015 by Arcturus Publishing Limited
26/27 Bickels Yard, 151–153 Bermondsey Street,
London SE1 3HA

ISBN: 978-1-78404-604-0
AD004452UK

Printed in China

Contents

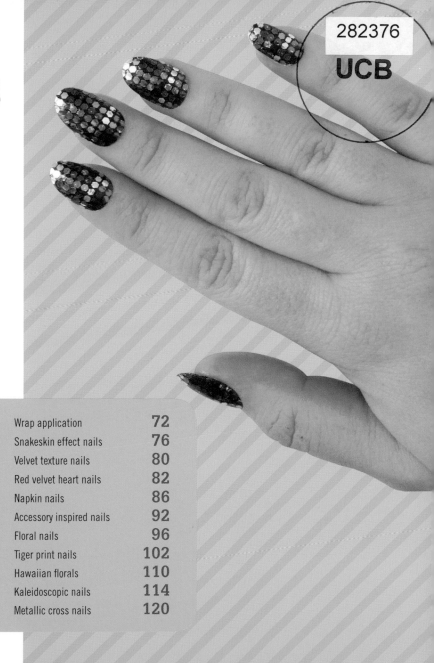

Introduction

Offering unlimited opportunity for expression, nail art has become increasingly popular in recent years, with designs ranging from subtle to extended and extravagant. The projects, tips and tricks contained in these pages will appeal to all those who are interested in creating a unique and flawless result, from the beginner to the professional manicurist.

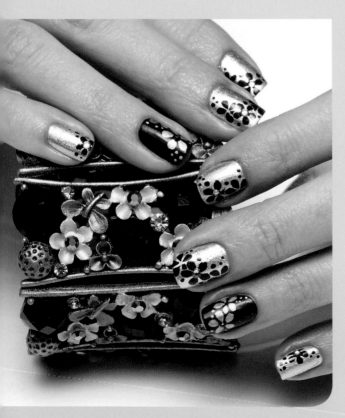

An affordable way to stay on trend, nail adornment through colour has evolved since henna and beeswax were used to stain the nail plate and signify social status over 5,000 years ago. Basic art began to make its way onto nails at the beginning of the 20th century, when subtle French and half moon manicures proved popular with actresses seeking a chic, well-groomed finish.

Nail lacquer colours have since developed, as has their texture and finish, and professional products such as gel polish, liquid and powder ('acrylic') can extend or enhance nails, allowing technicians to push the boundaries of design. From short to stiletto in shape, flat to 3D and multi-coloured in style, extended shapes can be created from the nail bed, and sculpting techniques, paints and tools used to translate imaginative ideas onto the tiny nail canvas.

While many nail professionals use this artistic ability and technical skill to create a requested design on nails, there are simple routes to nail art. Press-on nails or adhesive wraps with pre-printed designs offer a short-term solution, while nail stickers, textured products and decals can be added to enhance an existing design. The use of coloured nail stripers or a thin brush with polish is ideal for freehand or detailed work and a combination of skills can produce eye-catching results.

Recent years have seen an explosion of textured products for nails. Technicians have been known to use velvet, chains, beads and even napkins in a nail design. With an endless array of tools available to aid design both at home and in the salon, such as stickers, gems, dotters and special effect top coats, the only restrictions are imagination and skill. While nail colour and art are increasingly accepted in working environments, practicality and personal taste will often dictate the extent of the design.

Even apparently complex nail designs can be achieved by those with limited artistic prowess. In this book, leading nail professionals from all over the world have divided some of their favourite designs into a series of steps, so there is the opportunity for every individual to pick a style of nail art through which to express themselves.

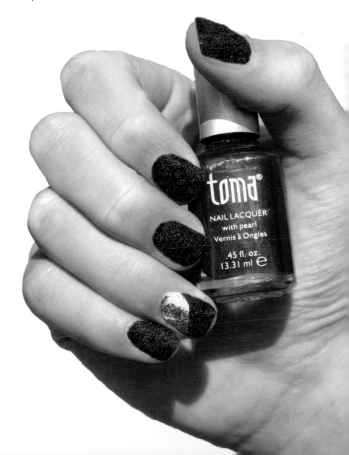

Facing page Nail technician Eva Darabos paints nails in silver metallic and black nail polish and embellishes them with crystals to accessorize alongside a jewellery item.

Right Sam Biddle paints nails in purple polish before dipping them in velvet particles for a textured finish. These nails feature a statement design in gold leaf on the ring finger.

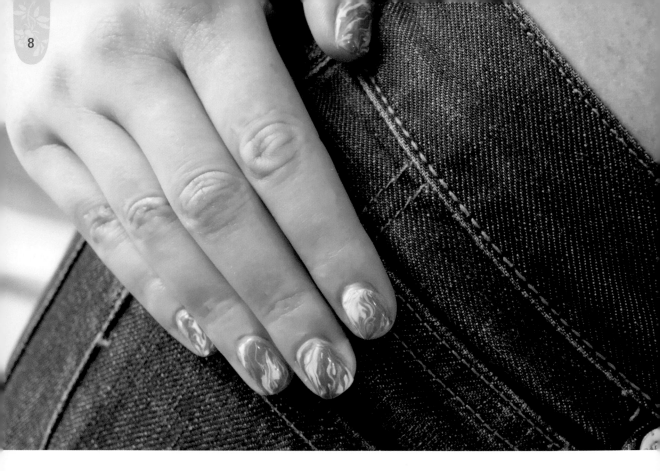

Getting started

Before commencing any nail project, it is important to prepare the nail. Good preparation maintains the health of the natural nail and ensures a smooth, shapely canvas on which to work. If preparation is skipped, nail products do not adhere well and can leave a poor nail finish, so even if professional nail technicians have little time on their hands, they will always perform basic nail prep.

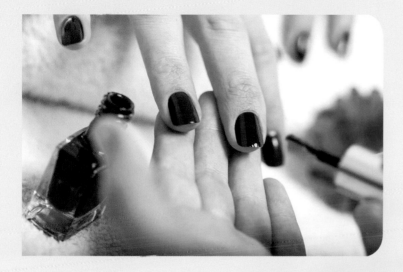

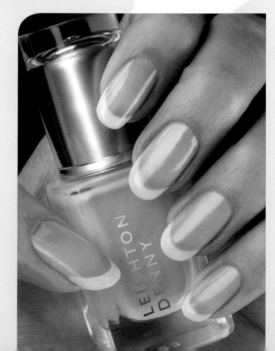

▲ A base coat is important before any polish colour is applied as it prevents the nail from staining and contributes to the longevity of the design. As a general rule, apply a base coat in one thin layer to the natural nail and allow it to dry before applying a thin coat of colour. When this first coat of colour is tacky or nearly dry, apply a second thin coat. Two thin coats of polish dry faster and last longer than one thick coat, which will simply peel off.

▶ When a nail design is finished, apply a thin layer of top coat and seal it at the edge of the nail to prevent chipping.

Preparation

Before you begin to decorate a nail, make sure that all the materials you need are to hand and you have enough time to complete your design.

Recommended kit

- Base coat
- Buffer
- Cotton pads
- Cuticle pusher
- Hand sanitizer
- Nail file
- Nail polish remover
- Paper towels

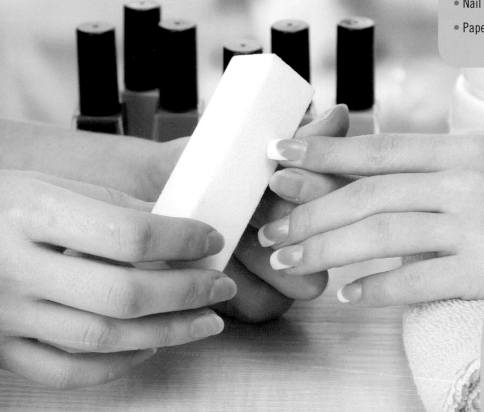

Top tip

If you have weak nails, use nail strengthener as a base coat.

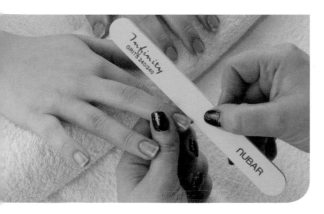

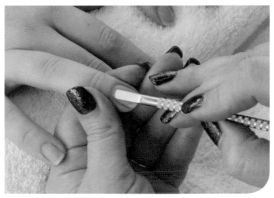

1 File the nails gently to the desired shape.

2 Tidy the cuticle area by pushing the cuticles away from the base and sidewalls of the nail, using a cuticle tool.

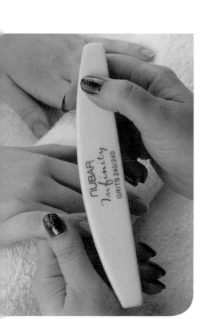

3 Use a buffer to lightly buff the nail plate and leave a smooth surface for application.

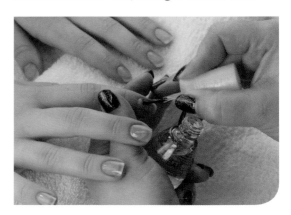

4 Apply a thin layer of base coat, leaving a 1mm gap round the edge of the nail. Allow to dry before beginning your design.

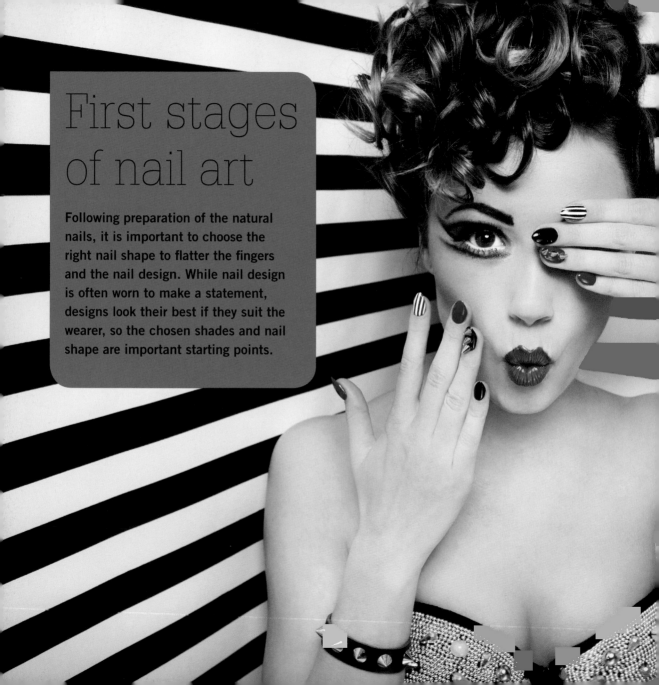

First stages
of nail art

Following preparation of the natural
nails, it is important to choose the
right nail shape to flatter the fingers
and the nail design. While nail design
is often worn to make a statement,
designs look their best if they suit the
wearer, so the chosen shades and nail
shape are important starting points.

Nail art terms

CUTICLE A layer of colourless, dead skin that clings to the nail plate and prevents bacteria from entering under living skin. Much of it is safely removed during a manicure.

FREE EDGE The end of the nail that extends beyond the tip of the finger.

NAIL BED The cells that support the nail plate.

NAIL PLATE The main part of the nail. It appears to be in one piece, but is constructed of layers which are attached to the skin at the tip of the finger.

SIDEWALL The skin either side of the nail plate. The sidewall acts as a barrier against bacteria and viruses. The term also refers to the area of nail free of the nail bed, extending beyond the skin sidewalls.

SMILE LINE The point where the nail bed ends and the free edge starts. It is a half circle that resembles a smile and it can be artificially created by a nail professional.

DECALS Any items, such as nail stickers, transfers or embellishments, that can be applied to the nail to enhance a design.

HALF MOON MANICURE A nail design where the natural 'half moon' of the nail plate (the curved, lighter area near the cuticle) is enhanced with a nail shade or pattern different from that of the rest of the manicure.

FULL MOON MANICURE A design where both the half moon and the free edge area of a nail are defined or painted in the same colour.

Free edge —
Smile line
Sidewall —
Nail bed
Nail plate —
Cuticle

Selecting the shape

The nail shape gives the foundation for a nail design. Nails and hands naturally vary in size and shape, from short fingers with short nail beds to long fingers with wide nail beds and every combination in between. Nail technicians can use professional products such as gel or acrylic to extend and sculpt an artificial nail to the desired shape, whether it be a long, pointy stiletto style nail or a 'lipstick' nail (a shape with a slanted or angular edge).

The most common nail shapes are square, oval, squoval, round and pointed, all of which are achieved by filing. The choice may depend on lifestyle as well as aesthetics – although the options with short and bitten nails are limited unless a nail technician enhances the short nail with professional products.

SQUARE The square nail is a popular choice for French manicures and can complement long nail beds and add length to fingers.

OVAL Oval nails offer a feminine look and can work with most nail beds.

SQUOVAL A squoval nail is an extremely versatile shape, offering the length of a square nail with the soft edges of an oval.

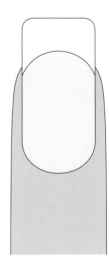

SQUARE File straight up the sides.

ROUND Round nails are less noticeable and are popular with men, as the shape mirrors the natural contours of the nail. A rounded shape can make large hands look slimmer.

POINTED Pointed shapes are highly adventurous and not very common. However, they can create length and offer an artistic shape in themselves.

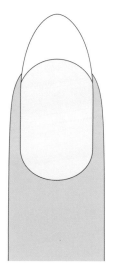

OVAL Use smooth, arching motions when filing to ensure a symmetrical finish.

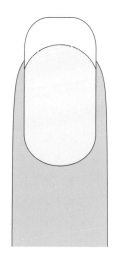

SQUOVAL File the nail into a square shape then file underneath the corners to soften.

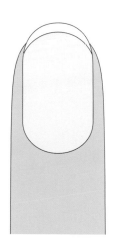

ROUND File the nail sidewalls outwards and round the edges into a curved shape.

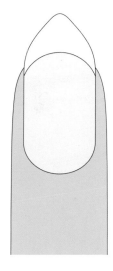

POINTED File diagonally from each sidewall to the middle point of the nail.

Choosing colours

Following fashion and seasonal trends as a way of deciding upon a nail colour is fun, but professional nail artists are trained to choose shades that suit a skin tone to achieve the best possible finish. Just as with clothes, certain nail colours can be unflattering against the skin and even give it a ruddy appearance, while others can make it look radiant.

Shorter nails benefit from pale shades which give the illusion of length, with vertical stripes of nail art for a subtle finish. People with longer nails can afford to be more experimental and draw attention to their nails with brighter shades and varied nail art.

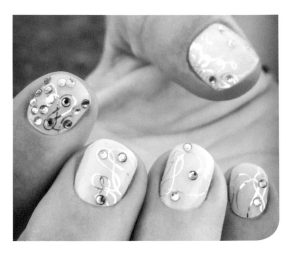

FAIR SKIN TONES

Most nail shades suit those with light or fair skin tones, although very pale skin may look sallow against extremely dark hues. Pinks, reds and lilacs work well to flatter fair skin.

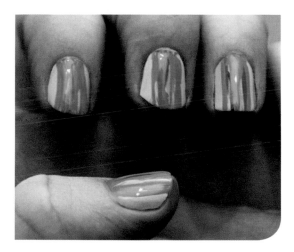

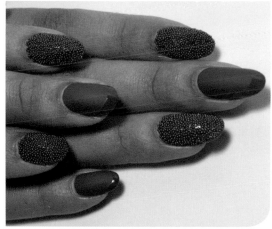

MEDIUM SKIN TONES

Nail art can be carried off well by those with medium skin tones, as varied prints and colours blend well with the skin. Metallic finishes and vibrant hues such as pink, orange, yellow and blue complement this tone; red, navy and dark purple should be avoided.

DARK SKIN TONES

Dark nail shades emphasize dark skin tones, and the warm hues of burgundy, red, green, gold and brown all look good. Tanned skin can also be complemented with lighter shades of blue and pink, but yellow-based colours are not recommended.

Essential tool kit

What do you need?

1 A natural-looking nail shade in pale pink or peach to suit your skin tone

2 A crisp white or milky white nail polish to create either a stark or natural looking white nail tip

3 A glossy top coat for a high-shine nail finish

4 A base coat in a clear or pale shade

5 An artist's brush, such as Leighton Denny Precision Brush, to remove smudges of polish and style smooth design shapes

6 A statement shade to suit your skin tone

7 Nail polish remover to take off existing polish and any smudges you make while you're working. You can also use it with a brush for design purposes

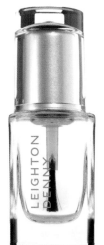

China Glaze Innocence

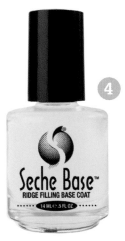

China Glaze White On White

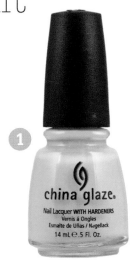

Leighton Denny Crystal Finish

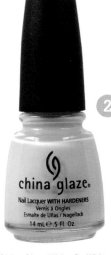

Seche Base

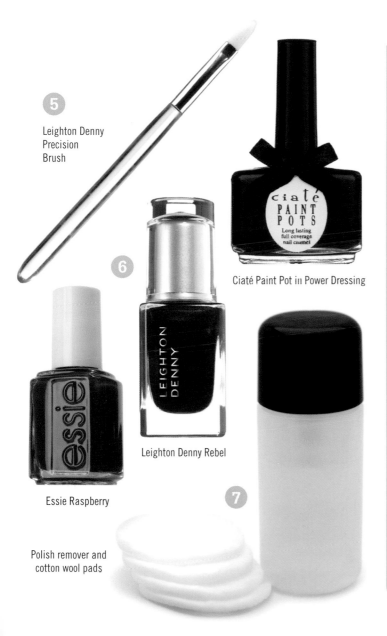

5

Leighton Denny
Precision
Brush

6

Leighton Denny Rebel

Ciaté Paint Pot in Power Dressing

Essie Raspberry

7

Polish remover and
cotton wool pads

ciaté
PAINT
POTS
Long lasting
full coverage
nail enamel

Five top tips for applying nail polish

1 Roll the polish bottle in your hands before application to give it an even consistency.

2 Hold back the skin on either side of the nail (the sidewalls) in order to reveal more of the nail area.

3 Apply the polish in three main strokes: in the middle, on the left of the nail, and then on the right.

4 Remember, two thin coats of nail polish last longer than one thick coat.

5 Never flood the cuticle with nail polish. Always leave a 1mm gap around the nail to prevent peeling and give the illusion of longer nails.

The essential nail art extras

1   A buffer to prepare the nail bed

2   False nails, with or without nail art additions

3   Nail glue or double-sided stickers for good adhesion of false nails

4   A nail art placing tool for easy pick-up of small decals

5   Instant effects polishes and top coats in a variety of shades and finishes

6   Complementary shades for subtle nail designs

7   Base and top coat to prepare and seal nail designs

8   Statement shades and funky polish colours

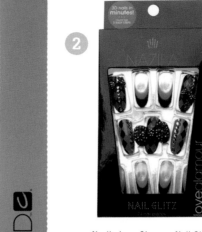

CND Girlfriend Buffer

Nazila Love Glamour Nail Glitz

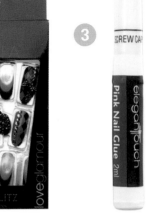

Elegant Touch Pink Nail Glue

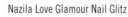

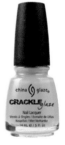

China Glaze Crushed Candy Crackle Glaze

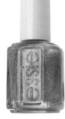

Essie Silver Bullions

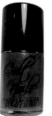

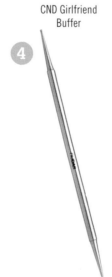

Nubar Nail Gem Placing Tool

Cult Nails polishes in Let Me Fly and Manipulative

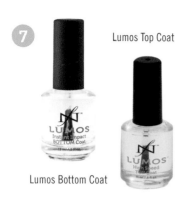

(7) Lumos Top Coat

Lumos Bottom Coat

(8) OPI Need Sunglasses

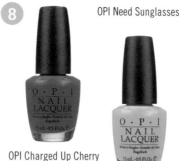

OPI Charged Up Cherry

Top tip

An alternative to a nail art placing tool is an orangewood stick or a pencil with a piece of Blu Tack on the end.

(9) Orly Instant Artist Large Dotter

(10)

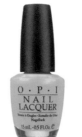

Art Club Striper in Pink Pastel

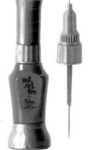

Nubar 2-way Hot Pumpkin Nail Art Pen

(11)

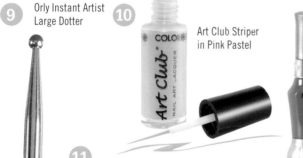

essie

Essie Corrector Pen

(13) EZArt stencils

(12)

Sponges

EZ Art Polish Stencils

ORLY

9 A dotting tool for easy creation of spots with polish

10 Polish stripers or a striper brush for lines and outlines

11 A corrector pen or brush and nail polish remover to get rid of smudges

12 A sponge for a mottled nail art effect

13 Stencils and transfers for flat, expressive nail art with minimal effort

Stick-on nails

Introduced as an economical response to the artificial nail craze of the 1980s, adhesive or 'stick-on' nail tips offer a quick fix for instant nail art. Ideal for short, unshapely or bitten nails, stick-on nails are favoured by session nail stylists who work on fashion shows or editorial photoshoots. To save time on set, stylists often pre-design the nails they need on plastic tips, then simply adhere and shape them to fit the models' nails just before the event.

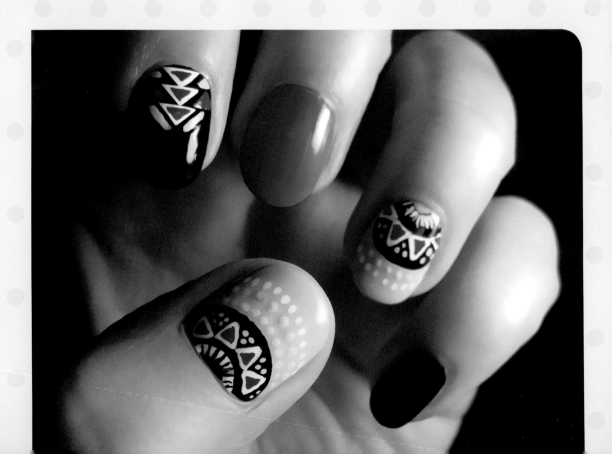

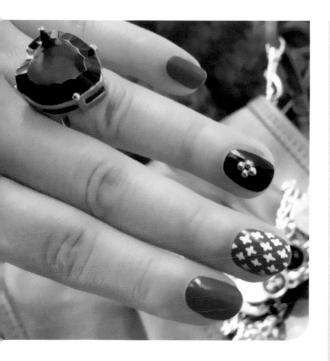

Five top tips for applying stick-on nails

1 Don't apply a base coat – simply buff the nail before application

2 Use nail glue instead of stickers for longer lasting nails

3 Press the artificial nail firmly onto the natural nail and hold for a few seconds until secure

4 To remove, gently lift the edge of the fake nail up and twist to the left and right slowly until it loosens

5 Avoid applying cuticle oil around the nail as this could weaken the adhesive

French style stick-on nails are popular, as are clear or pink-tinted tips for a natural look. Nail art and polish can be applied on top of these tips. In recent years, tips manufactured with pre-applied nail art have entered the mainstream as a solution for those less attuned to freehand nail artistry. A vast range of shapes, colours and designs includes styles to suit any personality or theme and serves as an ideal outfit accessory, to be applied simply with adhesive stickers or nail glue.

Above Stick-on nails in embellished and tweed designs by Susanne Paschke of Supa Nails.

Facing page Tribal-style stick-on nails handmade by Susanne Paschke of Supa Nails.

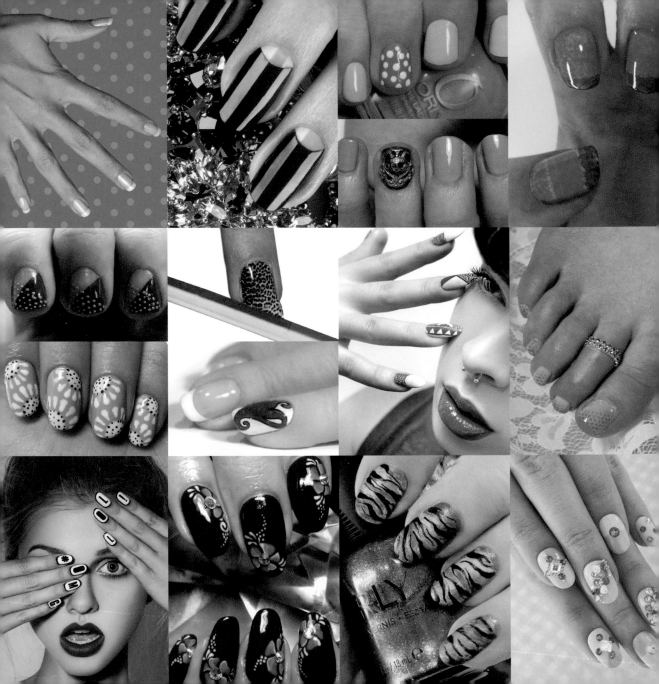

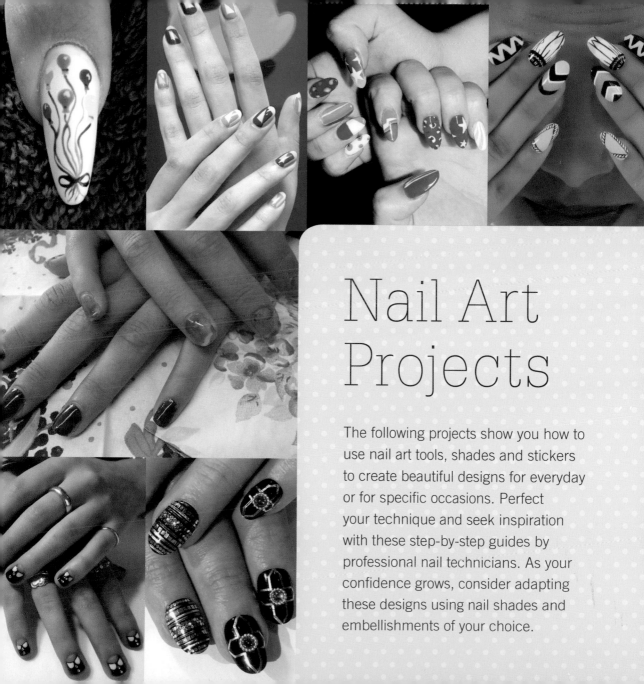

Nail Art Projects

The following projects show you how to use nail art tools, shades and stickers to create beautiful designs for everyday or for specific occasions. Perfect your technique and seek inspiration with these step-by-step guides by professional nail technicians. As your confidence grows, consider adapting these designs using nail shades and embellishments of your choice.

PROJECT: FRENCH MANICURE

The French manicure is a classic style designed to replicate the colouring of the natural nail. If done properly, it can make a short nail look longer and slimmer and can be tailored to suit any skin tone by using variations on the classic pale pink shade.

You will need

- Base coat
- Nail polishes in pale pink and white
- Top coat

An accurate, steady hand is required when painting a French manicure tip. Stencils, kits and false nails with pre-painted tips can all make things easier, but applying a white tip with a polish brush takes some practice. Use a thin artist's brush to improve accuracy and keep the look understated by following the smile line – the line between the main area of the nail and the nail tip. Keep the white tip in proportion to the size of your nail bed; short nails look best with a thin white tip, longer nails can afford a thicker tip.

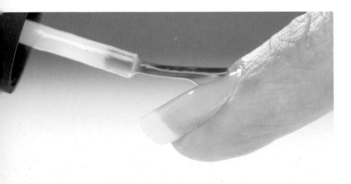

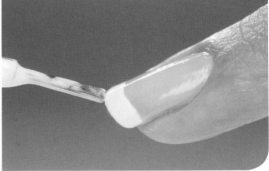

1 Apply a base coat to the nail, not forgetting the underside of the free edge. Apply one coat of pale pink nail colour while the base coat is still tacky.

2 Using a smooth, confident motion, paint a white tip and seal the free edge. Do not paint underneath the nail. Apply a second coat of white if desired.

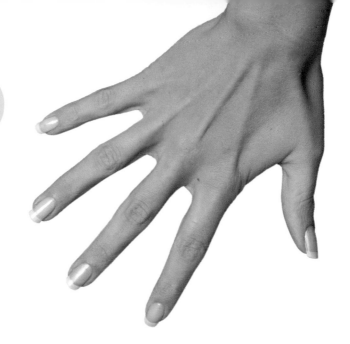

Top tip

Practise smooth, curved shapes with white polish on coloured paper before attempting the white tip on nails.

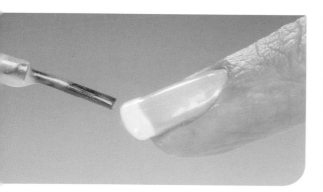

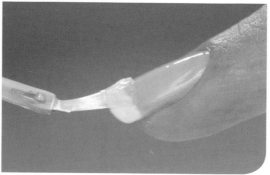

3 When the white tip is dry, sandwich it with a second coat of pale pink, painting under the nail and sealing the free edge.

4 Lock in the manicure with a glossy top coat, again painting under the nail and sealing the free edge. Allow to dry.

PROJECT: HALF MOON MANICURE
by Leighton Denny

A coloured nail with a naked half moon, or half moon in a contrasting colour, is popular in glamour advertising as it elongates the nail bed for a feminine look and epitomizes vintage style charm.

You will need

- Base coat
- Nail polish shade of choice
- Thin artist's brush
- Nail polish remover
- Top coat

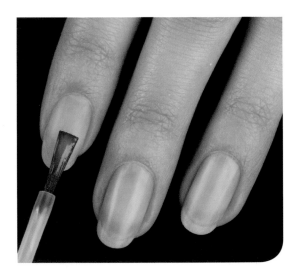

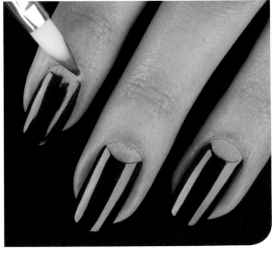

1 Apply the base coat, but leave the half moon area naked.

2 Apply two thin coats of your chosen nail shade and tidy the half moon shape using an artist's brush dipped in nail polish remover.

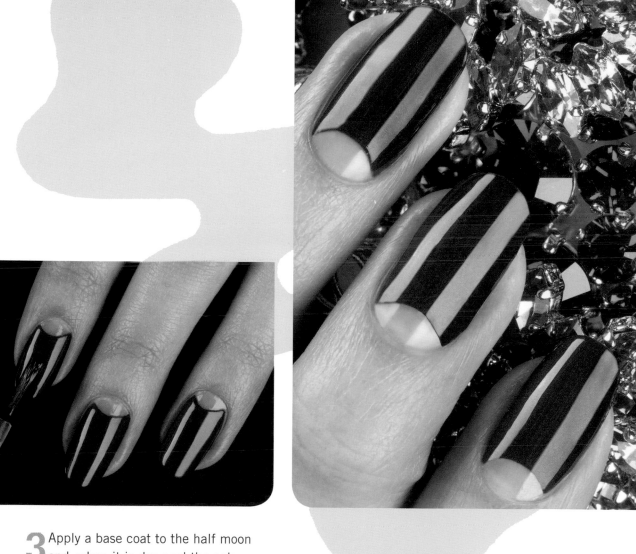

3 Apply a base coat to the half moon and, when it is dry, seal the colour with a thin application of top coat.

Image gallery

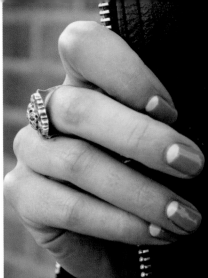

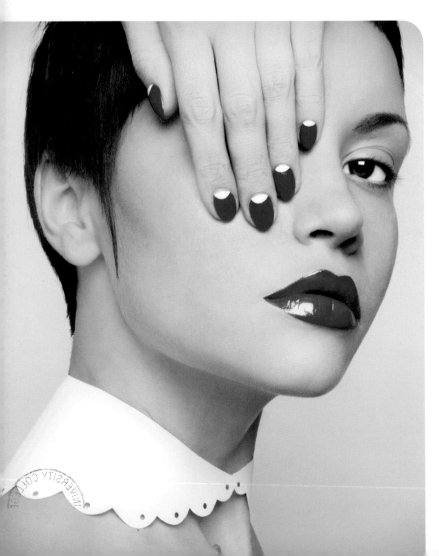

Above A colourful half moon manicure inspired by the sun breaking through a grey sky, by nail artists from Bio Sculpture Gel UK.

Left Striking scarlet nails in an almond shape, featuring a white painted half moon.

Below Nude and orange nails with a straightened half moon style, by Christina Rinaldi.

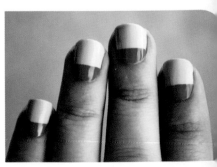

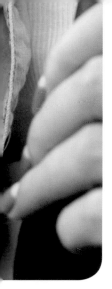

Right A striking combination of half moon manicure and French manicure styles with embellishment, by Ami Vega.

Below An edgy variation on the half moon manicure in grey and pink, by artists from Bio Sculpture Gel UK.

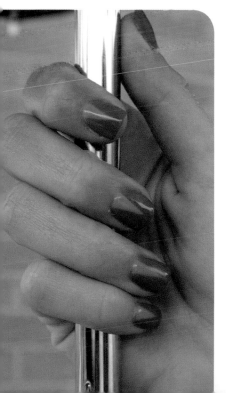

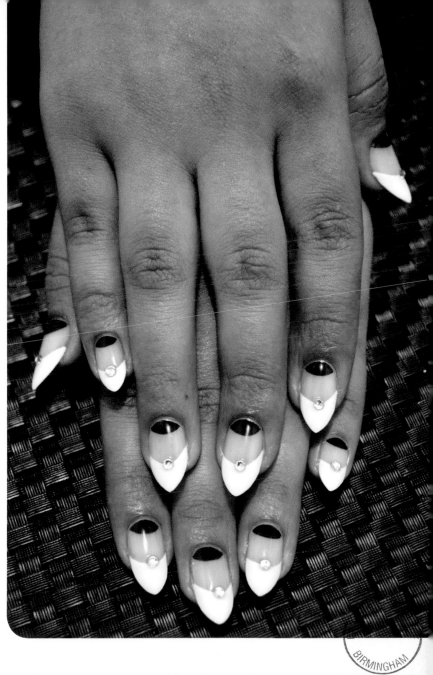

BIRMINGHAM

PROJECT: STATEMENT NAIL
by Leah Light

Rhinestones and small motifs add depth to a nail design. Easy to apply, they can be fixed with nail glue or placed on a wet top coat and left to dry.

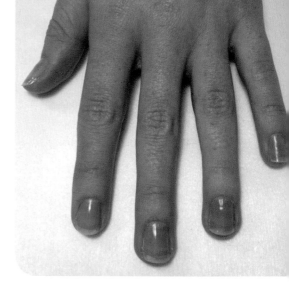

You will need

- Base coat
- Two contrasting nail polish shades
- Top coat
- Nail embellishment

1 After preparation, apply a base coat to the nails.

Shade suggestions

Cult Nails polish in Manipulative

Cult Nails polish in Let Me Fly on the ring finger

Nail Veil embellishment from Chronicle Stones

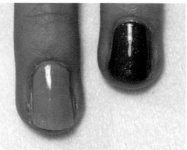

2 Paint a thin layer of the chosen statement shade on the ring fingernail and apply one coat of a contrasting or complementary shade to the remaining nails.

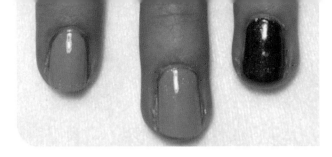

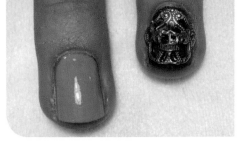

3 Apply a second coat of each colour to give full, even coverage. When dry, apply a top coat and cap the free edge.

4 Add another layer of top coat to the ring finger and, while it is still wet, place an embellishment on the nail and hold until the polish is dry.

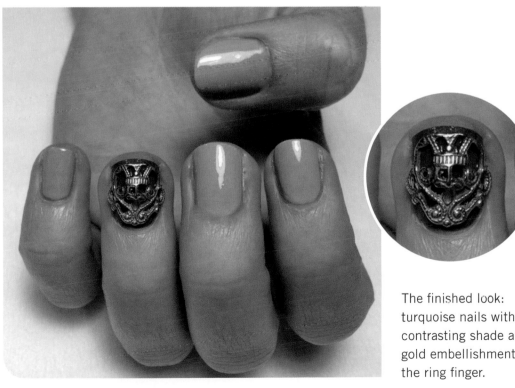

The finished look: turquoise nails with a contrasting shade and gold embellishment on the ring finger.

Image gallery

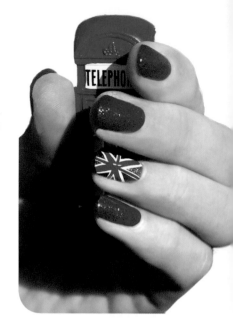

Right British-themed nails in scarlet with a hand-painted Union Jack on the ring finger, by Sam Biddle.

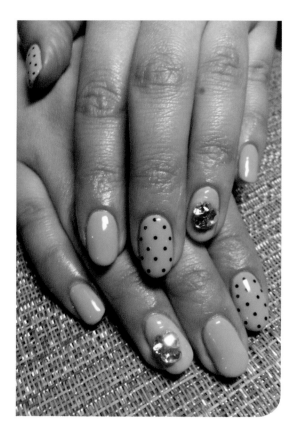

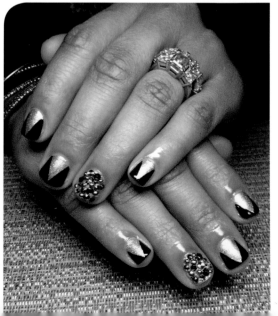

Above Natural nails painted in a delicate lilac shade with polka dots and embellishments on the feature nails, by Fleury Rose.

Right Gold, shimmery nails with a black hand-painted effect and crystal encrusted ring fingers, by Fleury Rose.

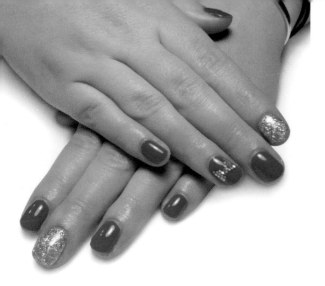

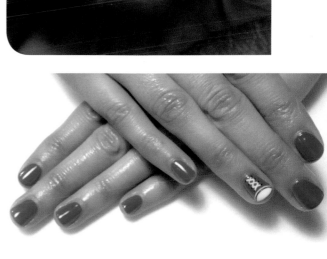

Above A neon-pink manicure with silver glitter feature nails and bow detailing on the ring finger, by Leah Light.

Right A bright nail design with two statement nails featuring decals and hand-painted dots, by Leah Light.

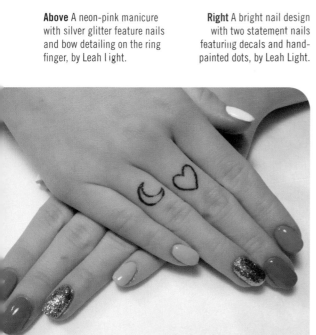

Left Nails in an assortment of bright shades with sparkly ring fingers, by Leah Light.

Above Neon-pink nails with a statement shoe design hand-painted on the ring fingernail, by Leah Light.

PROJECT: DOTTY ABOUT YOU
by Sam Biddle

Pretty and eye-catching, with a touch of 1950s charm, this dotted design for nails is simple and speedy to achieve. Create the look in three easy steps.

You will need

- Base coat
- Two nail shades
- White nail shade for dots
- Dotting tool or toothpick
- Top coat

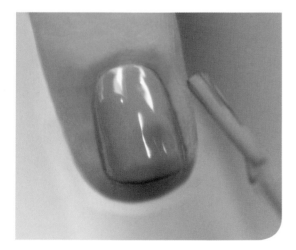

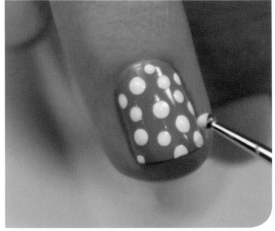

1 After an application of base coat, paint one of your chosen nail shades in two thin coats on eight nails, leaving the ring fingernails bare. Paint the ring fingernails a contrasting shade in two thin layers.

2 Dip the end of a dotting tool or small toothpick into white polish and randomly dot the ring fingernails.

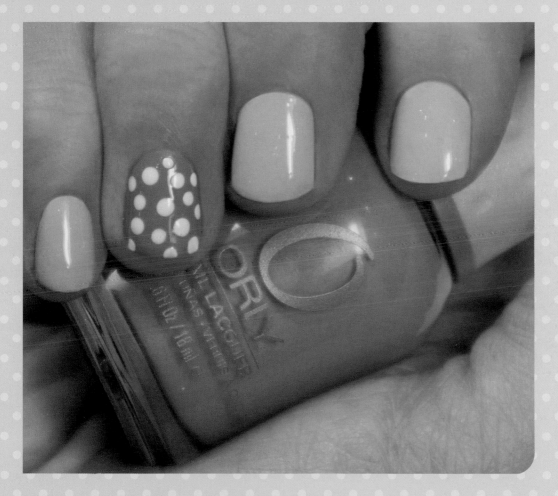

3 Allow to dry fully and apply a top coat, remembering to seal the free edge of the nail to prevent premature chipping.

Image gallery

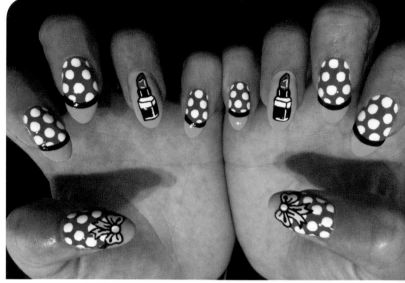

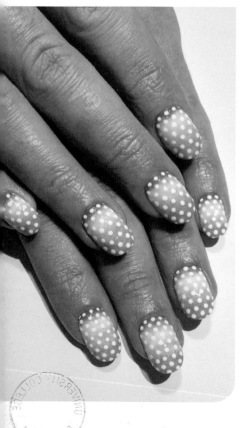

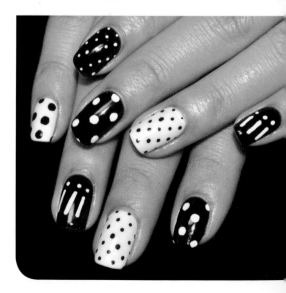

Above Playful polka-dot nails with hand-painted lipstick details on the ring fingers and bows on the thumbs, by Sophie Harris-Greenslade.

Left Rainbow nails created by sponging on a variety of colours; finished with white dots, by Sophie Harris-Greenslade.

Right Monochrome nails with varying sizes of dots and stripes, by Megumi Mizuno.

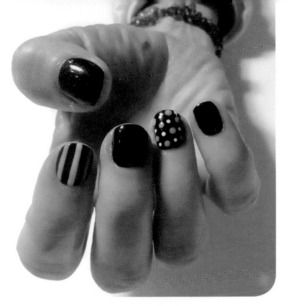

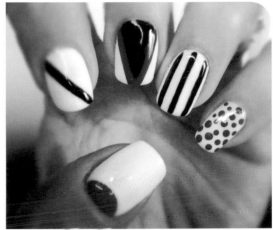

Above Deep purple nails with statement dots and stripes, by Leah Light.

Above right Nails with an assortment of stripes, dots and the half moon style, by Leah Light.

Right An eye-catching multi-coloured dot design, by Gemma Lambert, to complement the black base. Gemma has used a light sparkle polish on the remaining nails.

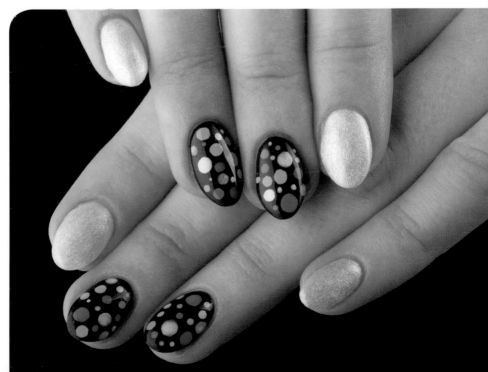

PROJECT: MULTI-TONE NAILS
by Carly Eva

Powerful, striking flat nail art can be achieved with colour experimentation. Multi-coloured nails suit the adventurous or those who find it hard to decide which shade to choose. The colours can be varied every season and with each manicure.

This simple project shows how to create a quick, colourful design on nails, using a sponge for a mottled polish finish.

You will need

- White nail polish
- Three nail polish shades of choice
- Sponge
- Nail polish corrector pen or artist's brush and nail polish remover
- Top coat

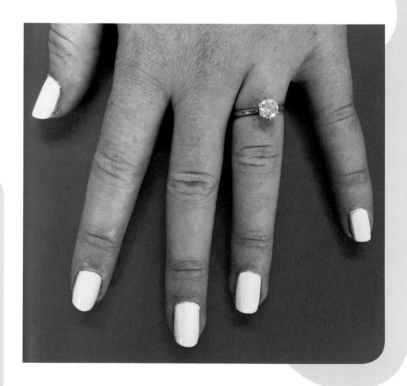

1 First, apply a base colour of nail polish in two thin layers.

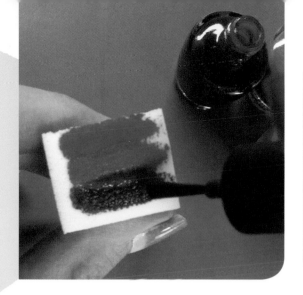

Shade suggestions

OPI Nail Lacquer in White Base

OPI Nail Lacquer in Formidably Orange

OPI Nail Lacquer in Riotously Pink

OPI Nail Lacquer in Seriously Purple

2 Next, apply three chosen shades to a sponge.

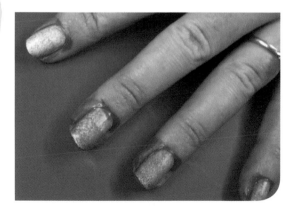

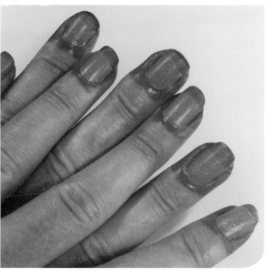

3 Press the sponge against the nail and roll it from left to right for full nail coverage.

4 Reapply the polish to the sponge and repeat for an intense look.

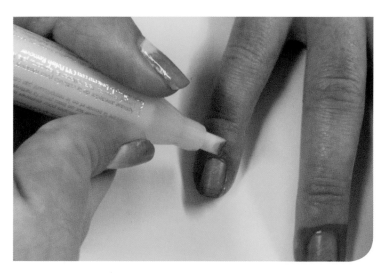

5 Remove excess polish with a corrector pen.

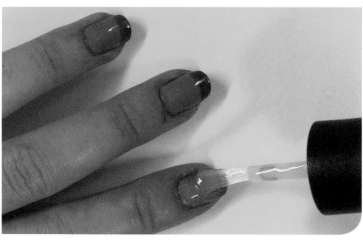

6 Apply a top coat to seal the design.

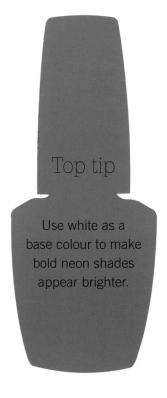

Top tip

Use white as a base colour to make bold neon shades appear brighter.

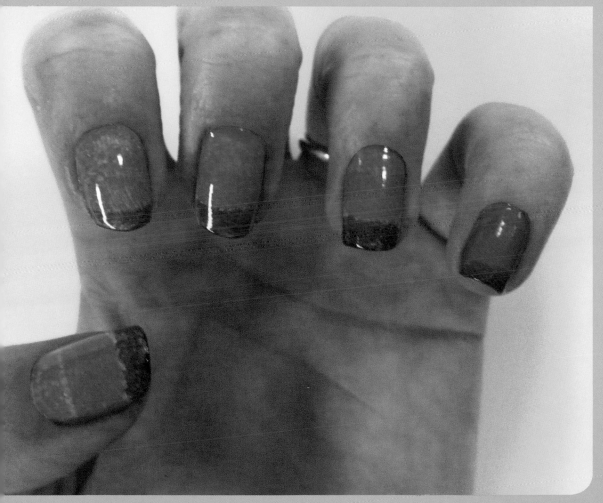

Striking, neon multi-tone nails created using
a sponging effect over a white base colour.

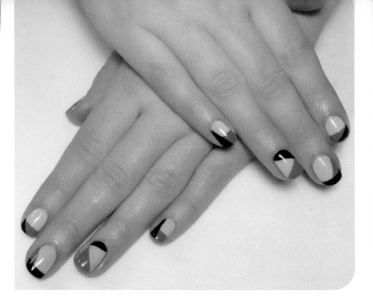

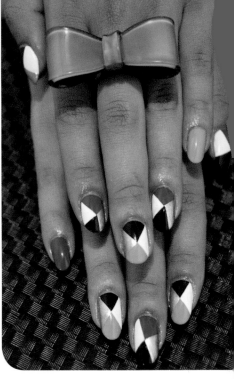

Image gallery

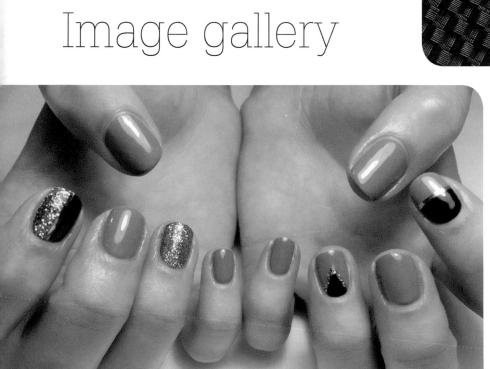

Above left Three contrasting shades are used in this geometric style, by Leah Light.

Above right
A kaleidoscopic nail design featuring triangular shapes in five shades which complement the model's ring, by Ami Vega.

Left Jade nails with random black and silver overlays and shapes, by Leah Light.

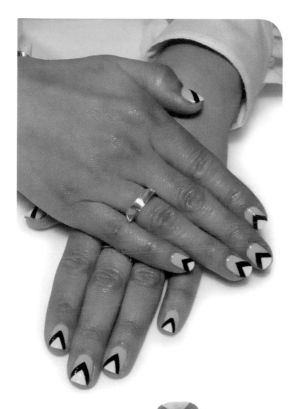

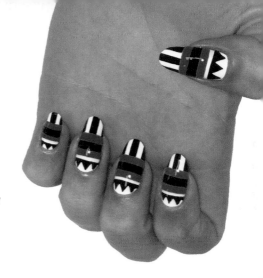

Left A striking chevron nail design in neon yellow, nude and black, by Leah Light.

Right An eye-catching tribal style nail look, by Sophie Harris-Greenslade.

Left Multicoloured chevron style nails, by Christina Rinaldi.

Right Varied geometric designs across all fingertips, featuring a neon yellow statement shade, by Ami Vega.

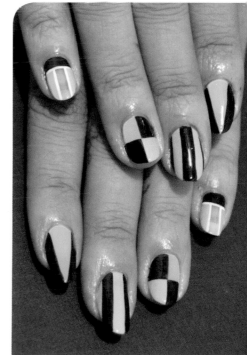

PROJECT: BIRTHDAY BALLOON NAILS
by Gemma Lambert

Create a balloon design on nails as a fun, eye-catching way to celebrate an occasion.

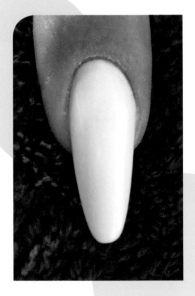
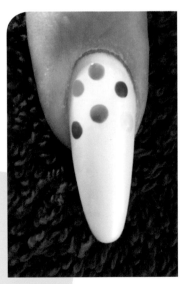
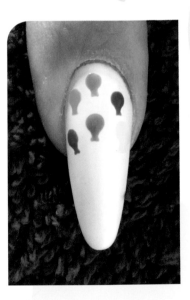

1 Shape nails to a point and apply the base coat followed by two coats of an opaque, white nail polish.

2 Using a dotting tool and an assortment of nail polish shades, add dots towards the cuticle end of the nail, allowing space in between them.

3 Using a thin brush or the smaller end of the dotting tool, extend the shape in the direction of the free edge of the nail to create the neck of the balloon.

You will need

- Base coat
- White nail polish
- Six bright shades of nail polish
- Black nail polish or striper
- Thin nail art brush and dotting tool
- Top coat

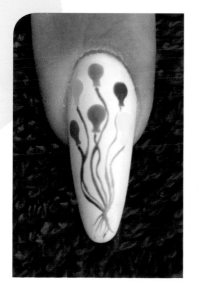 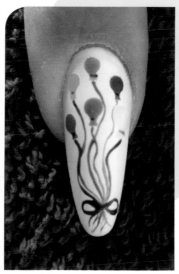 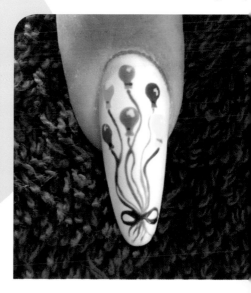

4 With black nail polish and a thin brush or a black nail striper, create the balloon ribbons, painting in a swirly shape towards the tip of the nail.

5 Add a bow to tie the painted ribbons together, and add dashes of black polish around the necks of the balloons to create a tied effect.

6 Use a thin brush and white nail polish to add a shine effect detail to the balloons. Allow to dry and then seal with a thin layer of top coat.

PROJECT: COLOUR-BLOCK NAILS
by Ami Vega

The design in this project uses the abstract shapes and bright colours associated with the 1960s Pop Art movement.

You will need

- Thin nail art brush
- Base coat
- Five pastel nail shades
- Top coat

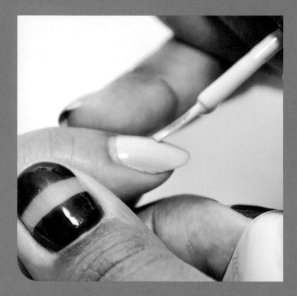

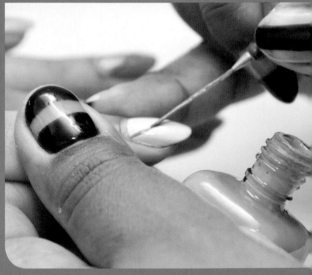

1 Apply a thin layer of base coat to all nails. Then apply two coats of pastel colour, using a different shade for each nail.

2 With a darker shade of each pastel colour, use a nail art brush to paint a diagonal line across the nail, from the cuticle to the free edge.

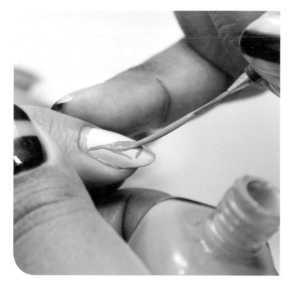

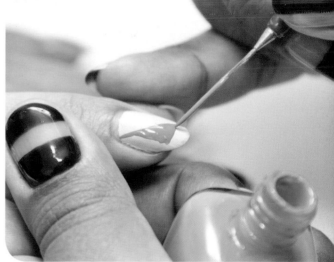

3 Outline the bottom part of the rectangle, below the diagonal line. Repeat on all nails, using a different colour on each one.

4 Fill in the bottom half of the rectangle you have outlined.

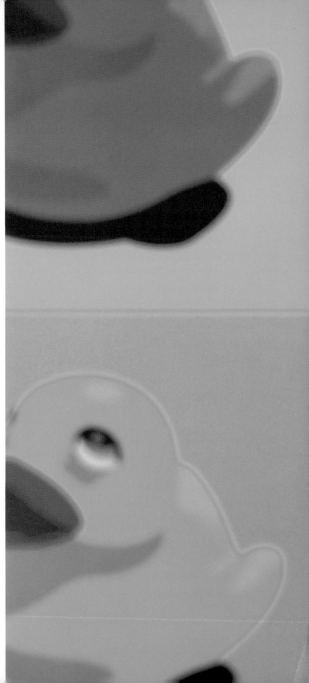

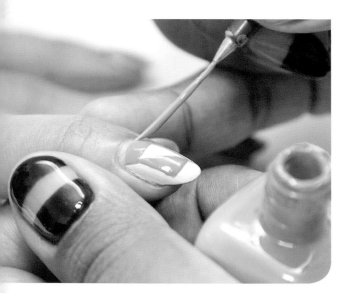

5 Create the top half of the rectangle on the other side of the diagonal line. This time, fill in the space around the shape (rather than inside it). Allow to dry, then apply a thin layer of top coat.

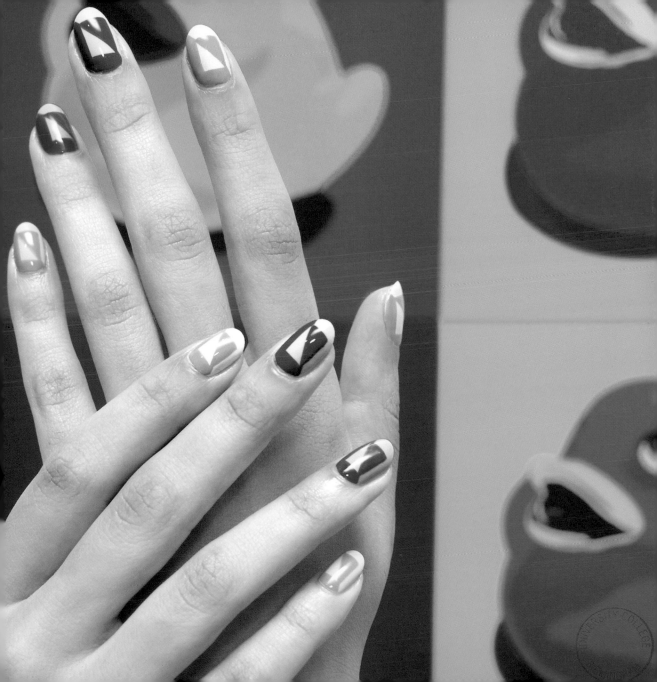

PROJECT: NEON LEOPARD PRINT NAILS
by Sophie Harris-Greenslade

Fun, quirky and surprisingly easy to create, these multi-coloured leopard print nails use contrasting bright colours and a random pattern. Colour placement does not have to be uniform and the black outline of the spots should vary for a realistic effect.

You will need

- White nail polish
- Four or five bright nail polish shades
- Black nail art pen or black nail polish and a thin artist's brush
- Top coat

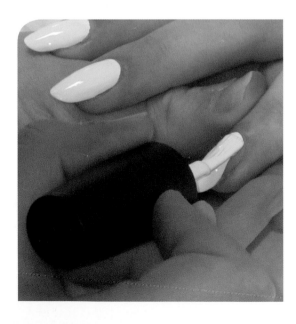

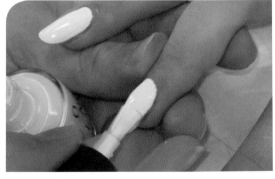

1 Apply one coat of white nail polish to all the nails.

2 Apply a second coat of white to the nails and cap the free edge; allow to dry.

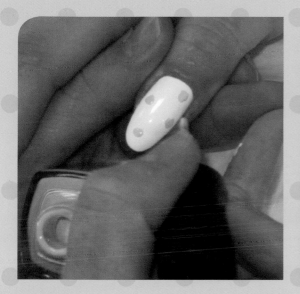

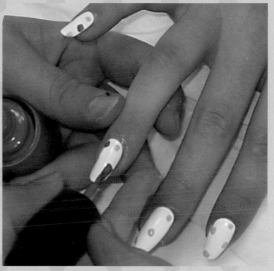

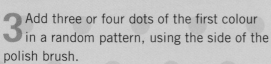

3 Add three or four dots of the first colour in a random pattern, using the side of the polish brush.

4 Add another three or four dots of a second, contrasting bright colour.

5 Add random dots of a third colour, remembering to keep the hand steady.

6 Add a fourth colour to the nails in a dotted pattern.

7 If there's space, add a fifth and final colour, filling in any large white spaces on the nail.

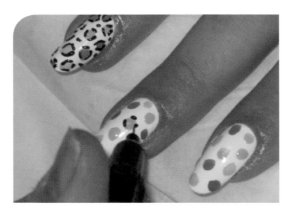

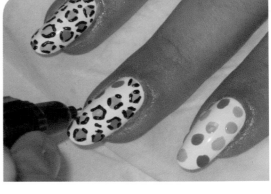

8 Using a black nail art pen, create a random sequence of three lines around each dot of colour. Start with a straight line at the top and curve the other two, leaving a small space between each one.

9 Continue around all the other dots of colour and add one or two dots or lines in any open white areas to stop the design becoming too uniform.

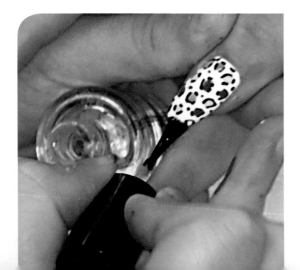

10 Repeat on the other nails and allow to dry. Seal with a top coat.

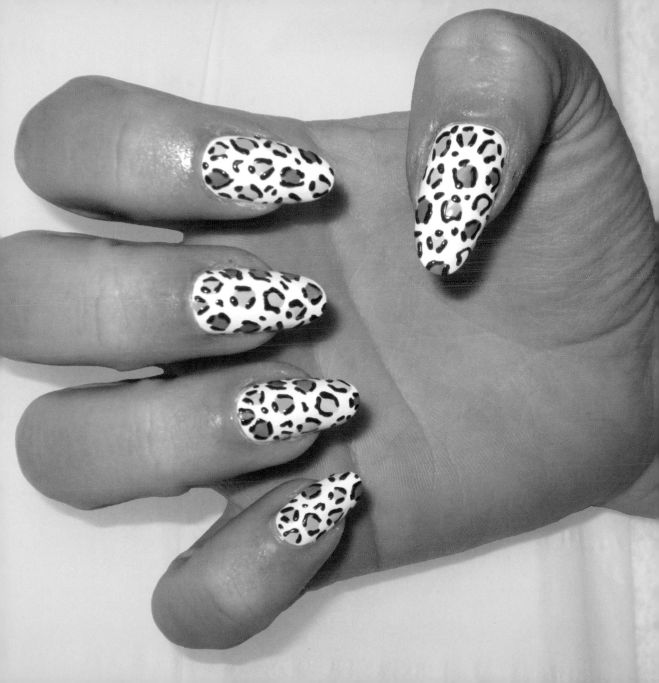

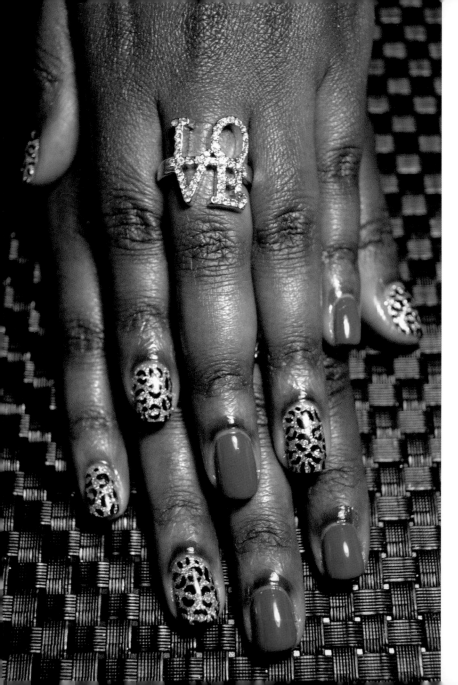

Image gallery

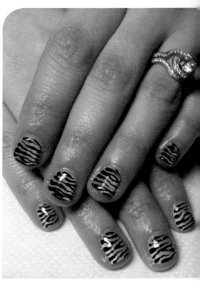

Above Nails inspired by tiger print, with hand-painted stripes on an ombré effect base, by Fleury Rose.

Left Squoval nails featuring a mixture of bright pink and glitter base shades, with freehand detailing in a leopard print style, by Ami Vega.

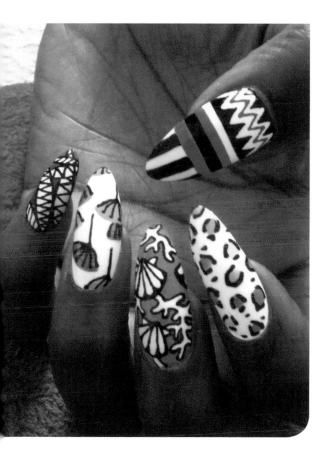

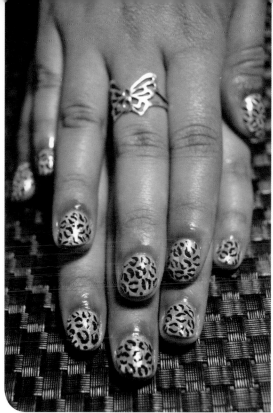

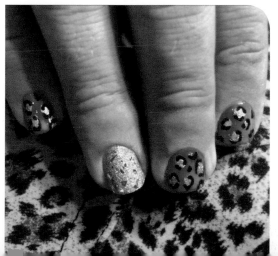

Above An assortment of bright, freehand nail designs in contrasting colours, including tribal patterns, sea shells and leopard print, by Sophie Harris-Greenslade.

Above right Neon multi-coloured nails with a leopard print effect, by Ami Vega.

Right Leopard print nails with a feature fingernail, by Christina Rinaldi.

PROJECT: TRIBAL NAILS
by Ami Vega

Tribal nail designs combine geometric patterns and bright, contrasting colours. The beauty of this style of nail art is that there is no limit to the number of colours you can use. It is a popular choice for people with a little more time to spend, a steady hand and some degree of patience, as each colour must be dry before you paint around it, to avoid smudging and colour bleeding.

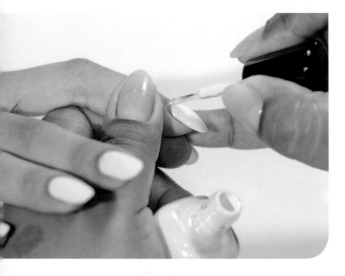

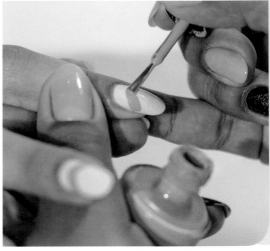

1 Apply a base coat followed by two thin coats of a yellow nail shade.

2 Create a 'V' shape in the middle of each nail using grey polish.

You will need

- Base coat
- Nail polish shades in yellow and grey
- Black nail striper or black nail polish and a thin artist's brush
- White nail striper or white nail polish and a thin artist's brush
- Top coat

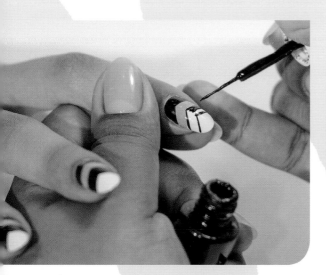

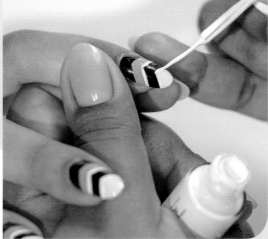

3 Fill in the space below the 'V' with a black nail striper and create another 'V' shape above the first one.

4 Outline the top black 'V' with a white striper and leave to dry.

A model shows oval nails with varied designs, including a rope effect and a striped tribal style pattern, using four shades of nail polish.

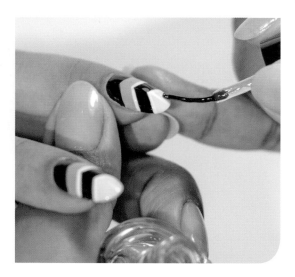

5 Apply a top coat to seal the design and give a glossy finish.

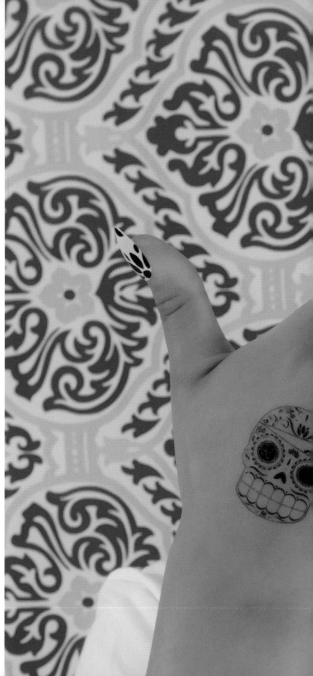

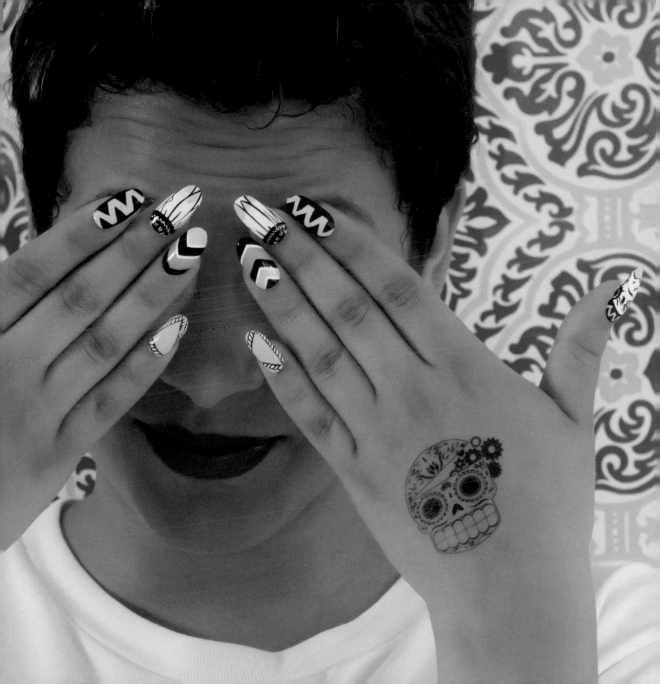

PROJECT: CROSSOVER POLKA-DOT NAILS
by Christina Rinaldi

This crossover design combines street style with popping colours and a twist on the half moon manicure. Achieve a quirky look by choosing a dark shade as the main colour and a bright, contrasting shade for the dots. Although this style requires precision, it is quick to do.

You will need

- Base coat or a translucent, pale nail shade
- Dark nail polish shade
- Dotting tool or thin artist's brush
- Bright nail polish shade
- Top coat

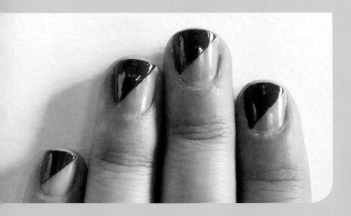

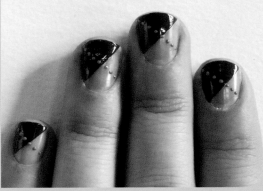

1 After an application of base coat or a pale nude shade, apply your chosen colour in a diagonal line from the corner of the half moon out towards the free edge. Apply two coats of polish to the upper half of the line and allow to dry.

2 Using a dotter and polish or striper in a contrasting colour, create a line of dots in the opposite direction from the other side of the half moon towards its opposite free edge.

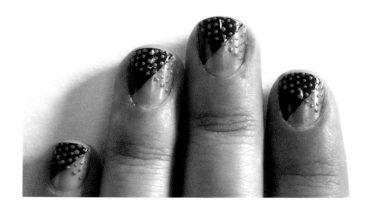

3 Using the first line of dots as a guide, apply further dots in a slightly angled direction upwards towards the free edge of the nail. Repeat on all nails and apply top coat when completely dry.

Nude and teal nails with a contrasting neon dotted pattern give a simple yet striking effect.

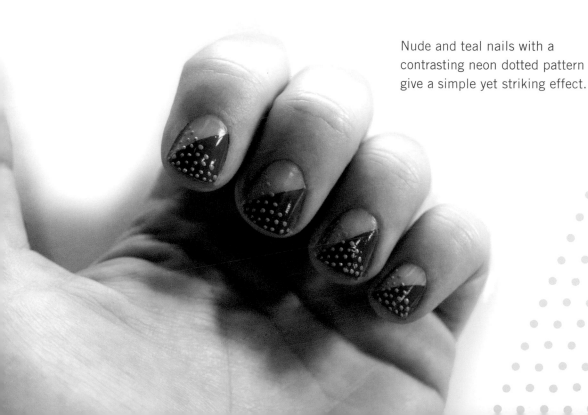

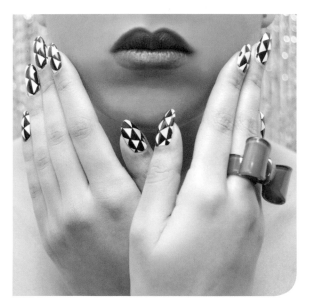

Left Almond-shaped nails with a monochrome design and a touch of mint green, by Ami Vega.

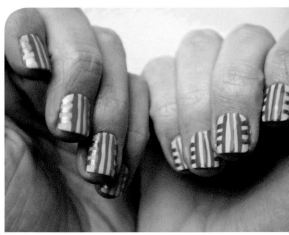

Image gallery

Below left A stylish black manicure with random white and gold detailing, by Christina Rinaldi.

Below right An extension of the half moon manicure with a dotted effect, by Christina Rinaldi.

Above Nails with a coral and gold stripe effect, by Christina Rinaldi.

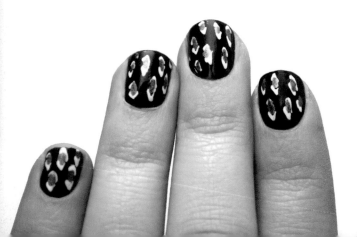

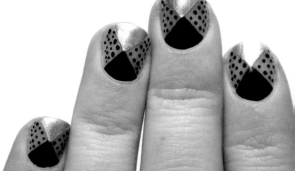

Below A modern take on the half moon manicure, with a triangular 'moon', in two striking shades, by Sophie Harris-Greenslade.

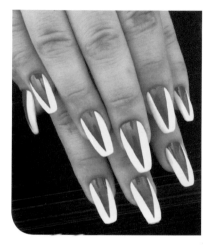

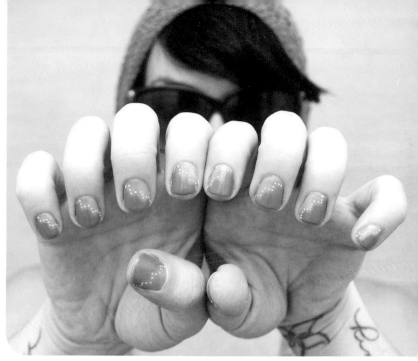

Below A floral manicure with a gradient design on the statement nail, by Christina Rinaldi.

Above A bright step-style design with dotted detailing, by Christina Rinaldi.

Below A matchstick inspired manicure, by Christina Rinaldi.

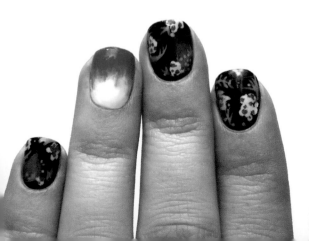

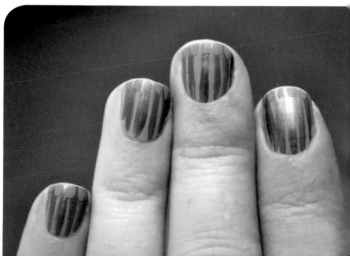

PROJECT: DAISY CHAIN NAILS
by Fleury Rose

Brighten up your nails with this fresh, floral, feminine design.

You will need

- Nail polishes in blue, yellow and black
- Thin art brush
- Dotting tool or small brush
- Top coat

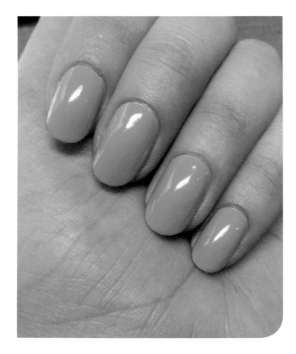

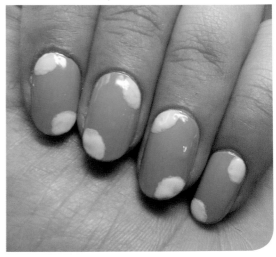

1 Apply two coats of sky blue polish and allow to dry for 5–10 minutes.

2 Using a pointed brush, dot yellow partial circles on opposite corners of each nail. Clean the brush.

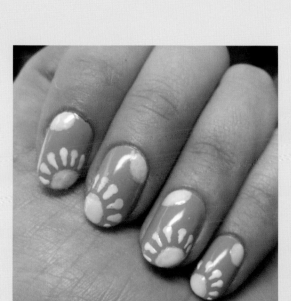

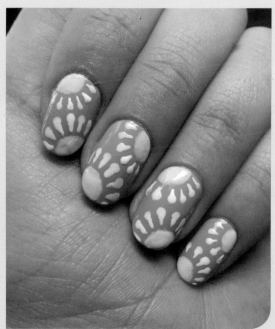

3 Use the brush and white nail polish to create the daisy petals. Dot the colour near the bottom yellow shape and drag outwards. Repeat around the bottom yellow shape on each nail.

4 Repeat Step 3 on the top yellow shape on all the nails.

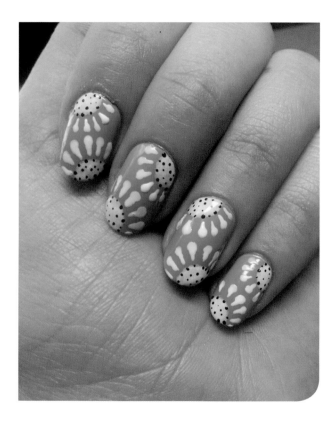

5 With a very small brush or dotting tool, add tiny black dots to the centre of the daisy design.

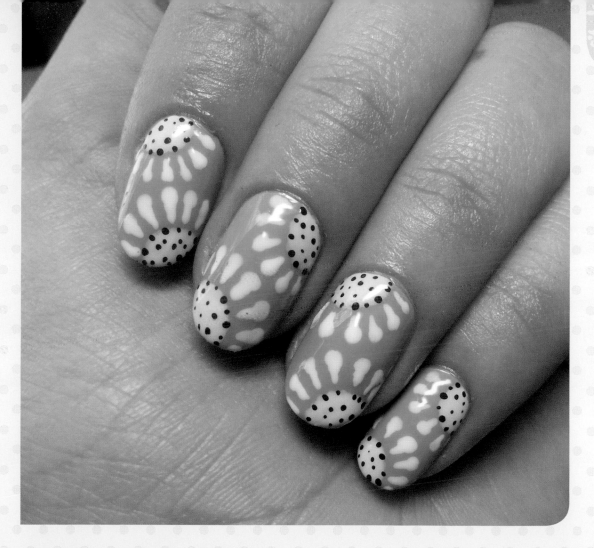

6 Allow the design to dry for ten minutes and seal with a top coat.

Image gallery

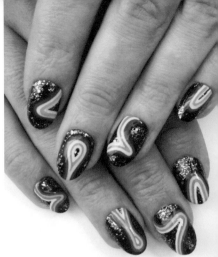

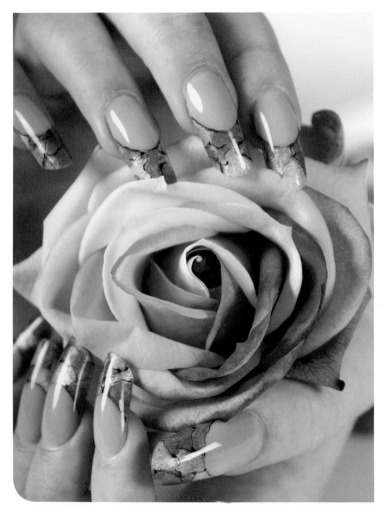

Above A galaxy themed nail art design with random rainbow freehand art, by Sophie Harris-Greenslade.

Left French style nails with a multi-coloured, marble effect tip, by Gemma Lambert.

Below Intricate hand-painted nail art in black and white, by Sophie Harris-Greenslade, created on square nails.

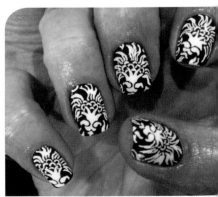

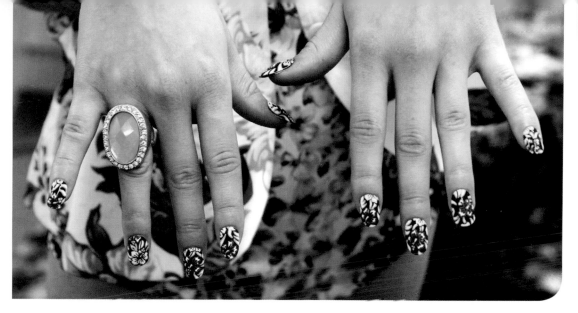

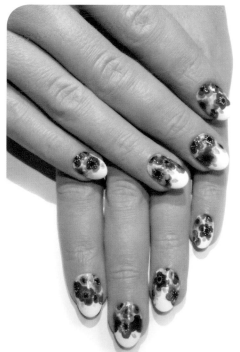

Above Hand-painted floral nails inspired by elements of the model's clothing, by Sophie Harris-Greenslade.

Right A 1960s style pink and purple pattern, painted freehand by Sophie Harris-Greenslade.

Left A striking floral nail design on an opaque white polish background, by Sophie Harris-Greenslade.

Right Bright yellow nails with a hand-painted lace effect, by Sophie Harris-Greenslade.

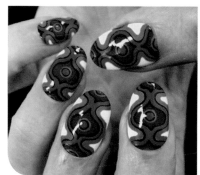

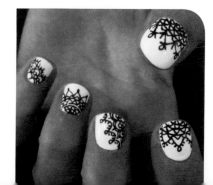

PROJECT: WRAP APPLICATION

Although they require some precision, nail wraps are easy to apply and remove, need no drying time and come in numerous designs to suit all trends and occasions. Once in place, they last for about a week and are popular with those who wish to make a statement with their nails by wearing a custom design or the latest patterns. They can be cut and shaped to suit the nail or to reflect nail trends, such as the half moon manicure.

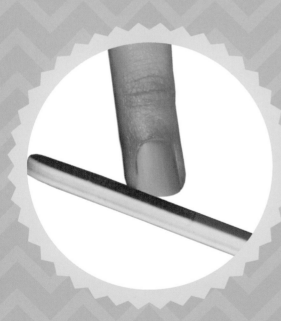

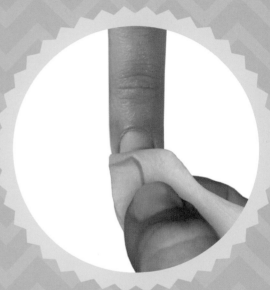

1 Push back the cuticle, then shape and file the nail edge. Gently remove the surface shine with a nail buffer or smooth nail file.

2 Clean the nail with a sanitizer or nail preparation wipe. Select the wrap size closest to that of the cuticle (trim to fit) then warm it between your fingers or with the hot air from a hairdryer before removing it from the backing sheet.

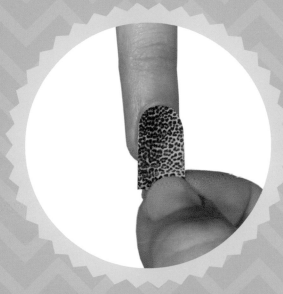

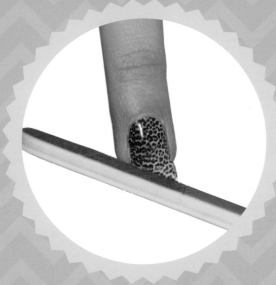

3 Place the wrap near the cuticle edge. Press firmly onto the nail and, working from the cuticle edge, apply pressure and smooth the wrap from the middle to the outside edges of the nail.

4 Smooth out any creases by lifting the wrap slightly and stretching it back over the nail before applying pressure and smoothing again. Extend the wrap over the free edge of the nail and file away any excess.

Wraps courtesy of Nail Rock

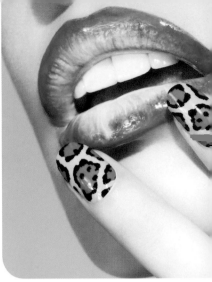

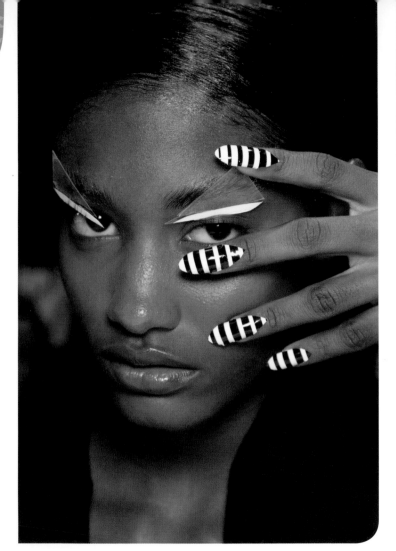

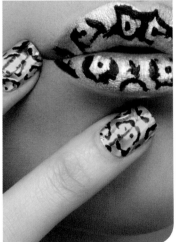

Above A model wears extended nails overlaid in black-and-white striped Minx for a Gareth Pugh collection. Nail look conceptualized by Marian Newman.

Image gallery

Facing page, top
Yellow cheetah print
Nail Rock wraps,
designed and applied
by Zoe Pocock.

Facing page, bottom
Gold giraffe print Nail
Rock wraps, designed
and applied by Zoe
Pocock.

Below Minx nail foils in
'Johnny' design layered
over the 'Lusion' style,
by Naja Rickette.

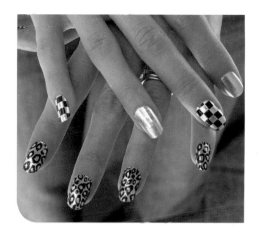

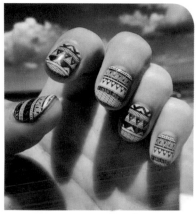

Above Leopard print
Minx nail foils on one
hand, contrasting with
silver and chequered
Minx on the other hand,
by Naja Rickette.

Above right Tribal style
monochrome nails, by
Naja Rickette.

Right Quail eggshell
effect Nail Rock wraps,
designed and applied
by Zoe Pocock.

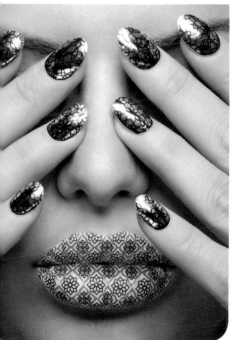

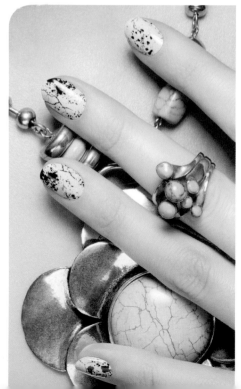

PROJECT: SNAKESKIN EFFECT NAILS
by Sam Biddle

Increasing demand for unique nails has led to greater experimentation with design and the products used. The opportunities are as endless as your imagination. Nails can be hung with feathers to produce a colourful look with an unusual texture. Small pieces of material, particularly lace, can look stylish on their own or act as a stencil for nail design. In this project, tulle is used as a stencil to create a fantastic snakeskin effect.

You will need

- Base coat
- Nude nail polish shade
- Tulle or netting
- Sponge
- Bright nail polish shade
- Top coat

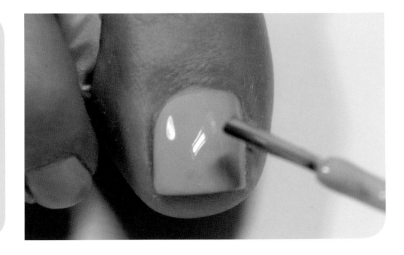

1 Prepare the nails by pushing back the cuticles and applying a good quality base coat. Apply a nude polish in two thin coats, using one that is as close to the skin tone as possible. Alternatively, try a darker, bolder base colour.

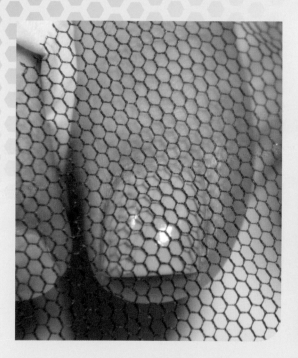

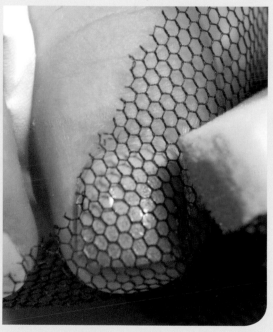

2 Place a piece of tulle over the dry polish and hold firmly.

3 Dab the sponge in a bright nail polish. Remove the excess, then press the sponge onto the tulle on the nail. You can dab all over or just on a section of the nail, depending on the look you want to achieve.

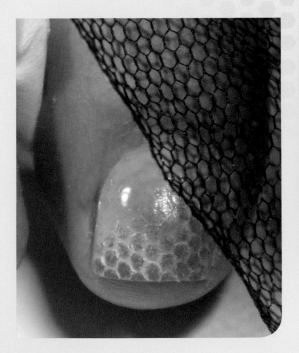

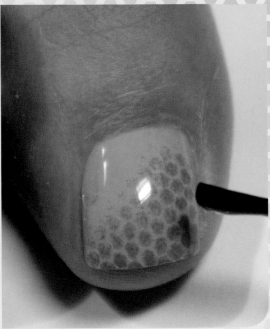

4 Gently peel away the tulle to leave a snakeskin effect.

5 Apply a layer of top coat to the nails and allow to dry.

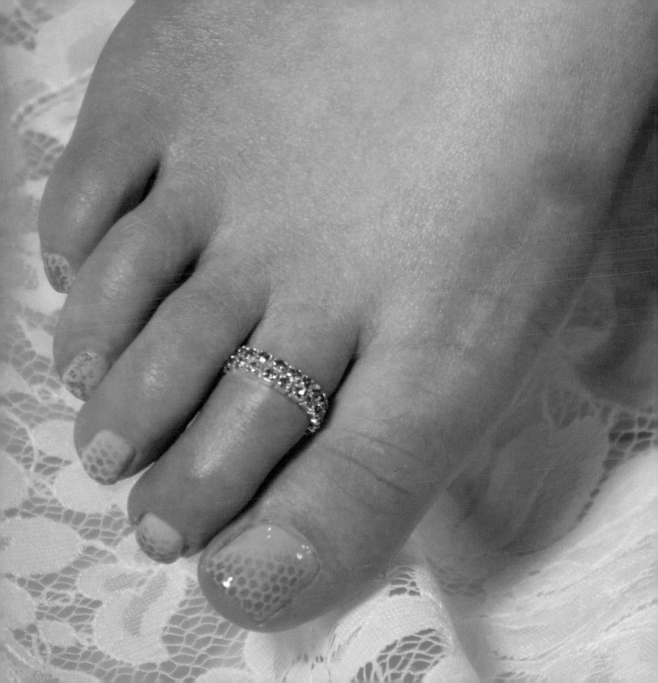

PROJECT: VELVET TEXTURE NAILS
by Sam Biddle

This project experiments with using texture. The nails are painted a purple shade then dipped in purple velvet particles for a textured finish. These nails feature a statement design in gold leaf on the ring finger.

You will need

- Base coat
- Nail polish shade of choice
- Gold leaf
- Velvet particles or Velveteen
- Top coat

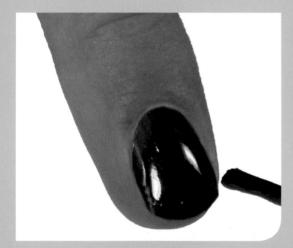

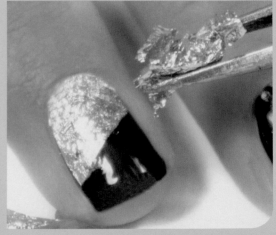

1 Apply a base coat and two coats of your chosen nail polish.

2 While the polish is still tacky, apply gold leaf to the ring fingernail with tweezers. Seal with a top coat and allow to dry.

3 Working with one nail at a time, apply a layer of top coat and dip the wet nail into the bag of velvet particles. Gently press the velvet into the top coat, then take your finger out of the bag and leave the nail to dry for 30 seconds. Blow off the excess velvet.

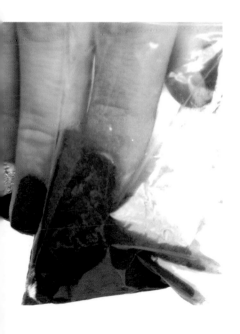

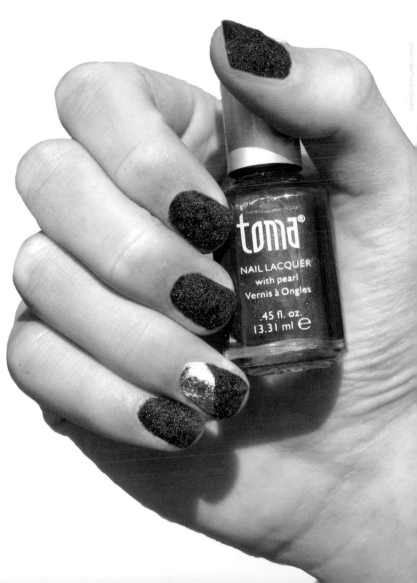

PROJECT:
RED VELVET HEART NAILS
by Sam Biddle

This statement nail with a textured element is a subtle way of celebrating St Valentine's Day.

You will need

- Base coat
- Nude or pale pink polish
- Thin brush
- White, red and black nail polishes
- Buffer
- Top coat
- Pencil
- Red velvet dustings or Velveteen
- Fan brush

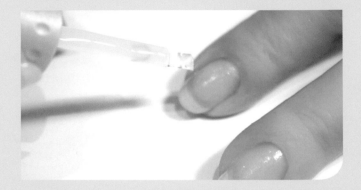

1 Apply a base coat to the nails, followed by one coat of nude or pale pink polish on all the nails except for the ring fingers.

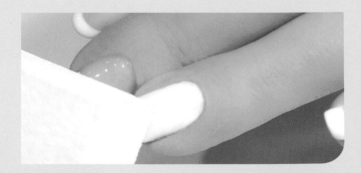

2 With a thin brush and white polish, create a white tip on the nails in French manicure style. On the ring fingers, apply two coats of white polish to the whole nail. Apply top coat to all the nails. When the ring fingers are dry, lightly buff the surface to create a matte finish. Do not buff the other fingernails.

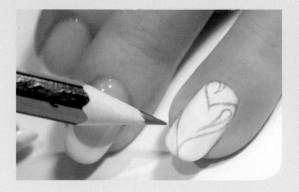

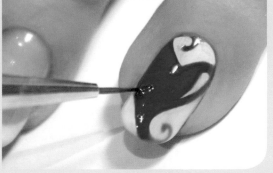

3 On the ring fingers, draw a heart design on the white polish using pencil. The pencil marks can be erased if you make a mistake.

4 Dip a thin brush in red polish and fill in the heart shape.

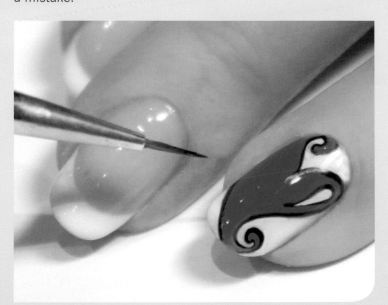

5 Enhance the shape by outlining it using black water-based nail paint or polish.

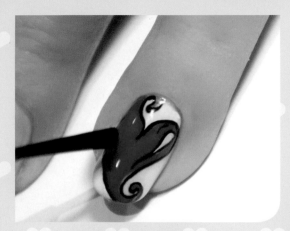

6 Allow the nails to dry fully and apply a layer of clear top coat to all of them.

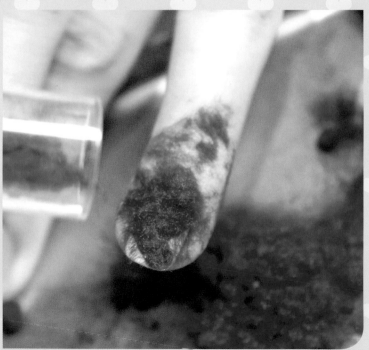

7 When the ring fingernails are dry, use a brush to apply another layer of top coat to the heart shape only. Sprinkle red velvet over these nails while they are wet.

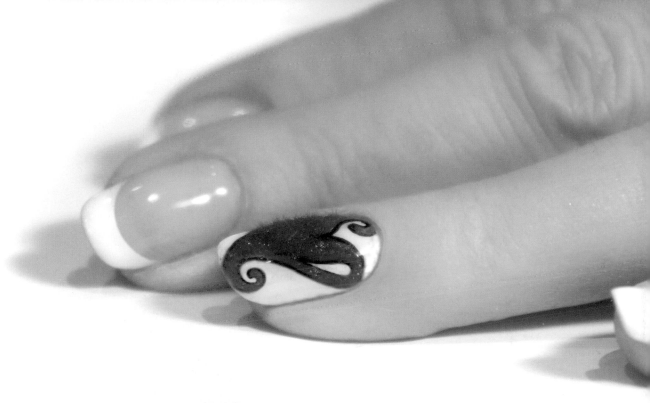

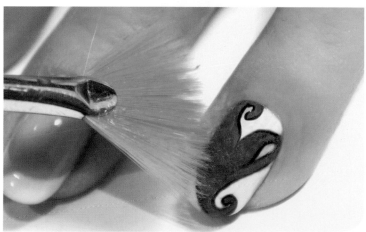

8 Leave the ring fingernails to dry for 30 seconds before removing any excess velvet with a fan brush.

PROJECT: NAPKIN NAILS
by Denise Wright

Use the printed patterns on napkins to create quick, striking designs. This style is ideal for seasonal occasions and people who are less at ease with freehand and intricate designs. It involves cutting patterns from a napkin and incorporating them into nail work.

You will need

- Base coat
- Napkin of choice
- Nail scissors
- Top coat
- Tweezers
- Nail file
- Nail glue

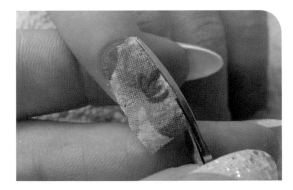

1 While the base coat is drying, cut the napkin to approximately the right size to fit the nail. Do not apply at this stage.

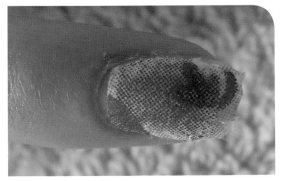

2 Trim the napkin neatly around the cuticle and sidewalls, but keep the length.

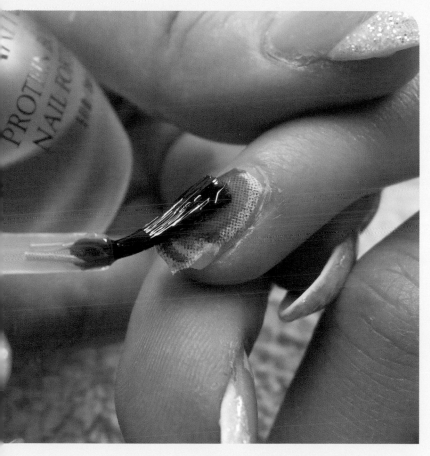

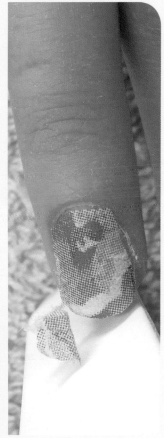

3 Apply a top coat directly over the base coat. While the polish is still wet, place the napkin piece over it and hold on to the nail – use tweezers if necessary. The top coat will seep through the napkin, forming a seal. While the top coat is still wet, apply another layer over the napkin design.

4 When dry, cut and file the excess napkin until the free edge of the nail is met.

Top tips

- Apply coloured polish after the base coat, if desired, to strengthen the design.

- Always split the layers of the napkin and only apply the top layer with the design to the nail, otherwise the paper will be too thick for the top coat to seep through.

- Apply an additional layer of top coat for a smooth finish.

- If stick-on nails are used, complete the application of the napkin on these nails before affixing them to the natural nail.

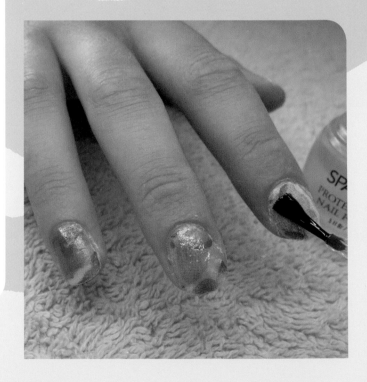

5 Repeat on all nails and seal the free edge with top coat or nail glue to prevent the napkin from peeling.

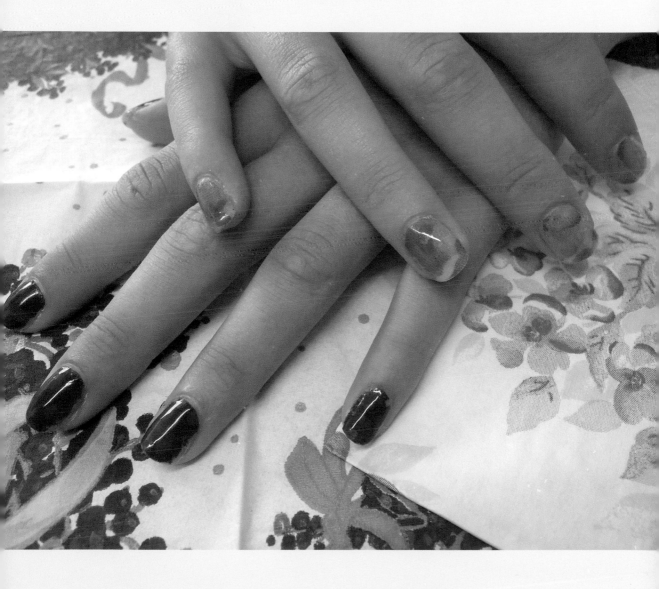

Image gallery

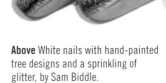

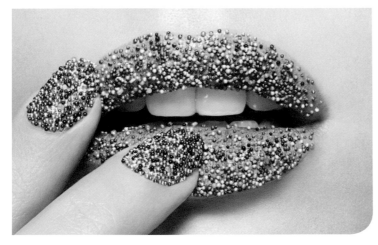

Above White nails with hand-painted tree designs and a sprinkling of glitter, by Sam Biddle.

Left The multi-coloured 3D Caviar Manicure™ by Ciaté.

Below Jet black nails with gold embellishments in a halo manicure style, by Sophie Harris-Greenslade.

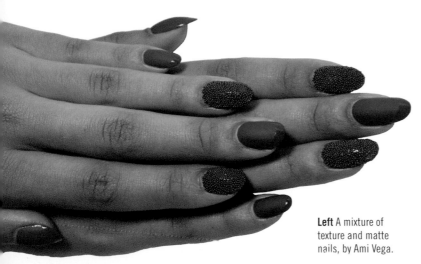

Left A mixture of texture and matte nails, by Ami Vega.

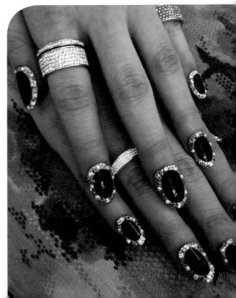

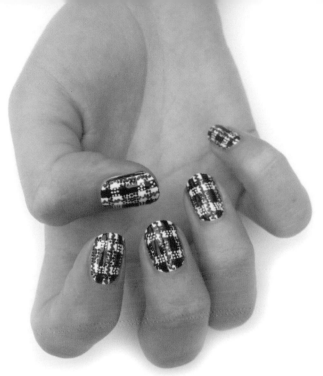

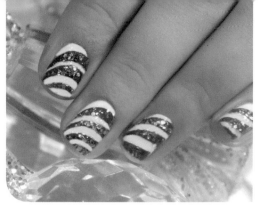

Left Hand-painted tartan print nail design, by Sophie Harris-Greenslade.

Below left Extended almond-shaped nails with a delicate pink shimmer gradient and featuring a gold butterfly embellishment, by Megumi Mizuno.

Above Short white nails with a festive red glitter effect reminiscent of a candy cane, by Sam Biddle.

Below Nail art inspired by Christmas knitwear, painted freehand in festive shades of red, blue and white, by Sophie Harris-Greenslade.

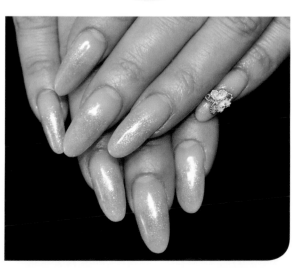

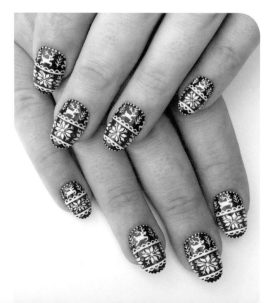

PROJECT: ACCESSORY INSPIRED NAILS
by Eva Darabos

This project shows how
to complement statement
jewellery items with a chic
nail design.

You will need

- Base coat
- Silver metallic nail polish
- Black nail polish
- Thin brush
- Crystals and diamantés
- Top coat

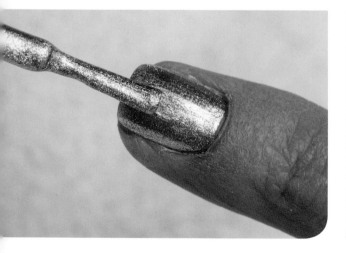

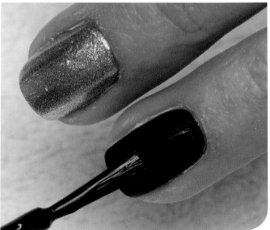

1 Apply base coat followed by two thin layers of silver metallic nail polish on all the nails except the ring fingers.

2 Apply base coat followed by two thin coats of black nail polish to the ring fingernails. Allow to dry for at least two minutes.

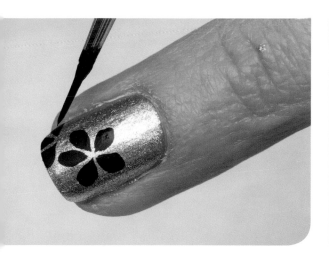

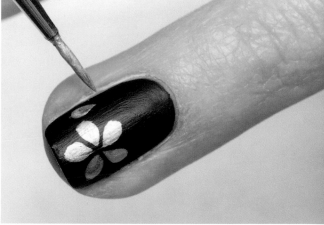

3 Dip a thin brush with a pointed end into the black nail polish and create flower designs on each of the silver nails. Change the position, size and number of flowers across these eight nails.

4 Repeat step 3 on the ring fingernails, this time using the silver nail polish.

Top tips

- Use shades such as silver, black, white, red, blue or rose that offer a timeless, classic effect.

- Consider using artist's acrylic paint for nail designs as it dries more slowly than nail polish, allowing for greater workability.

- Experiment with top coats such as matte, glitter, gloss or holographic for a super-eye-catching nail finish.

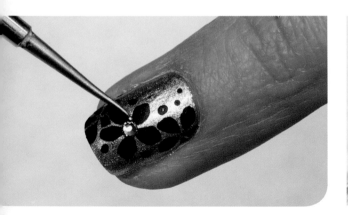

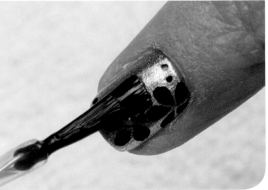

5 Complete each nail design by adding some dots around the flowers. Add a dab of top coat in the centre of some of the flowers and affix a crystal or diamanté. Allow the design to dry.

6 Apply a thin layer of top coat to all the nails and allow them to dry.

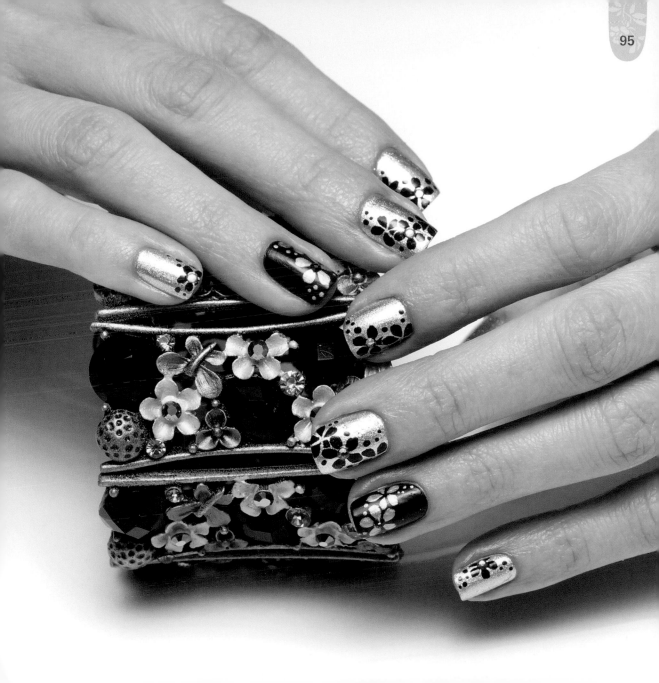

PROJECT: FLORAL NAILS
by Gemma Lambert

Jazz up plain, polished nails with a fancy hand-painted floral design.

You will need

- Base coat
- Two thin nail brushes
- Three coloured nail polishes
- White nail polish
- Top coat
- Crystals or diamantés

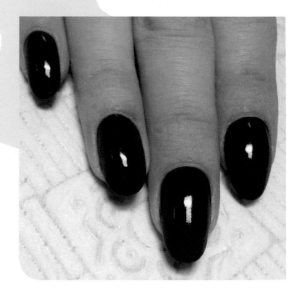

1 Apply a base coat and two coats of one of your chosen shades of nail polish. Allow to dry.

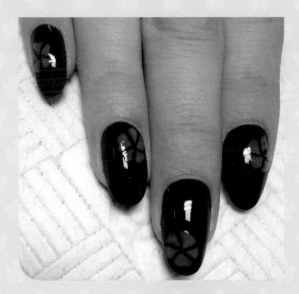

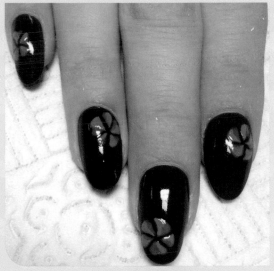

2 Using a thin brush and a lighter shade of polish, create five triangular petal shapes on each nail. Leave space between each shape and alter the position of the design on each nail.

3 When the petals are dry, take the third shade of polish and paint over half of each one.

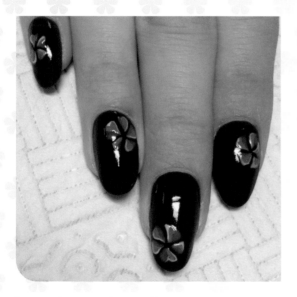

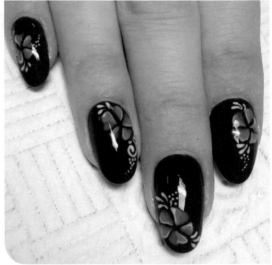

4 Using a fine brush dipped in white nail polish, add an accent to each of the petals along half of the top edge and down one side.

5 Continuing with the white shade, enhance your design with leaf effects as shown and add a cluster of small dots. Allow to dry thoroughly then apply a top coat. While this is still wet, add a diamanté or crystal to the centre of each flower.

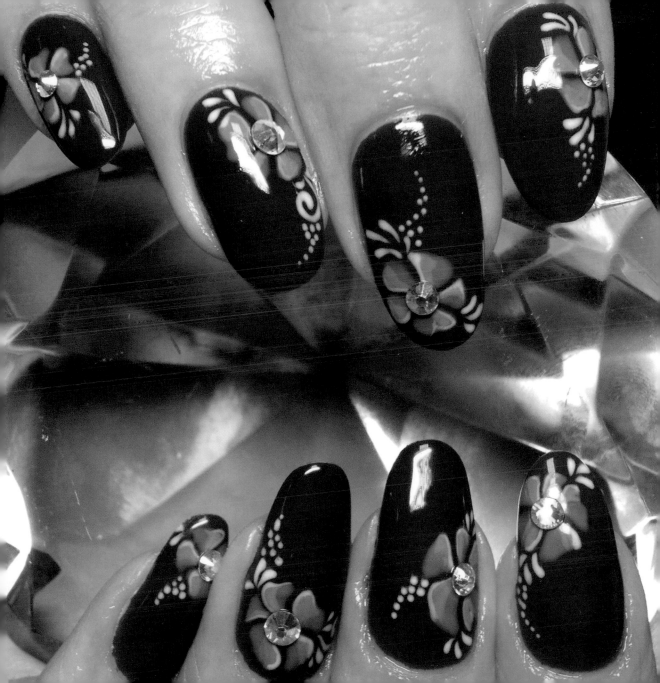

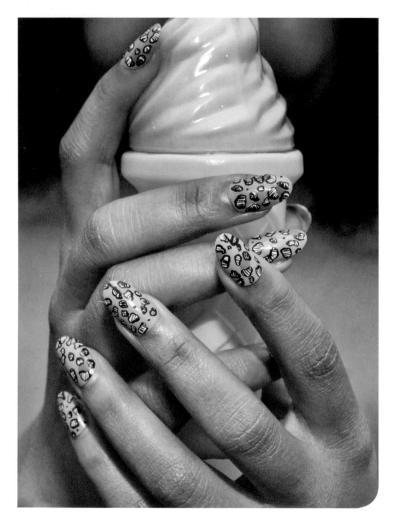

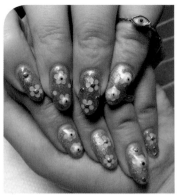

Above Sparkly nails featuring flowers and details inspired by a ring, by Fleury Rose.

Left Pretty pastel summer themed nails, by Ami Vega.

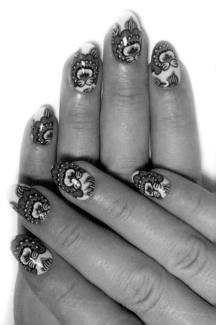

Image gallery

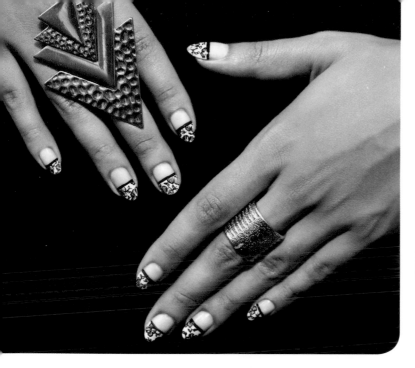

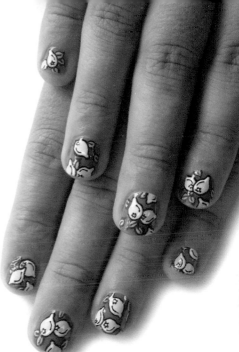

Above An elegant nail look, slightly influenced by the French manicure, featuring a timeless monochrome floral design painted freehand by Ami Vega

Above right A fruity freehand design in bright shades, by Sophie Harris-Greenslade.

Right A hand-painted paisley design on a colourful background, by Ami Vega.

Left Oval nails with a bright floral design randomly positioned across them, by Sophie Harris-Greenslade.

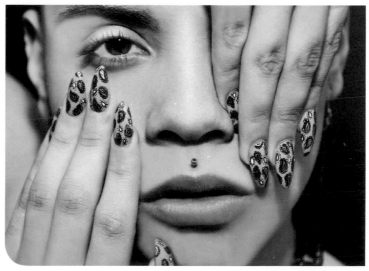

PROJECT: TIGER PRINT NAILS
by Sam Biddle

Complement an animal print fashion item with a tiger nail style for a coordinated look.

You will need

- Base coat
- Orange glitter nail polish
- Water-based acrylic or craft paints in cream, gold and black
- Thin nail art brush
- Matte top coat

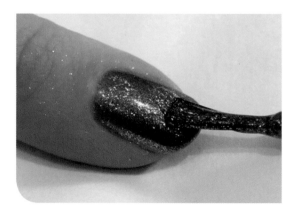

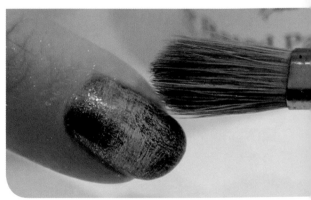

1 Apply a base coat, then paint the nails with two thin coats of orange glitter nail polish. Allow to dry.

2 Using a dry brush, such as an old make-up brush, dust a cream water-based acrylic paint or craft paint towards the centre of the nail.

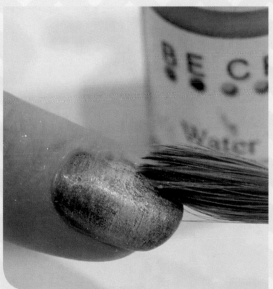

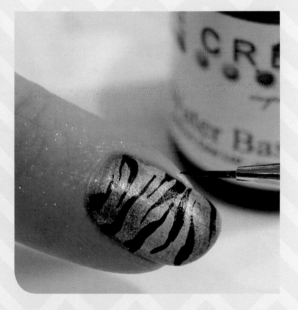

3 Use a gold water-based paint to brush over the cream shade lightly so that all three shades can be seen.

4 Use a thin nail art brush and black nail polish or acrylic paint to paint tiger stripes. Give the stripes a wide base and a tapered point. Work down the nail, alternating the direction of the stripes. Allow to dry.

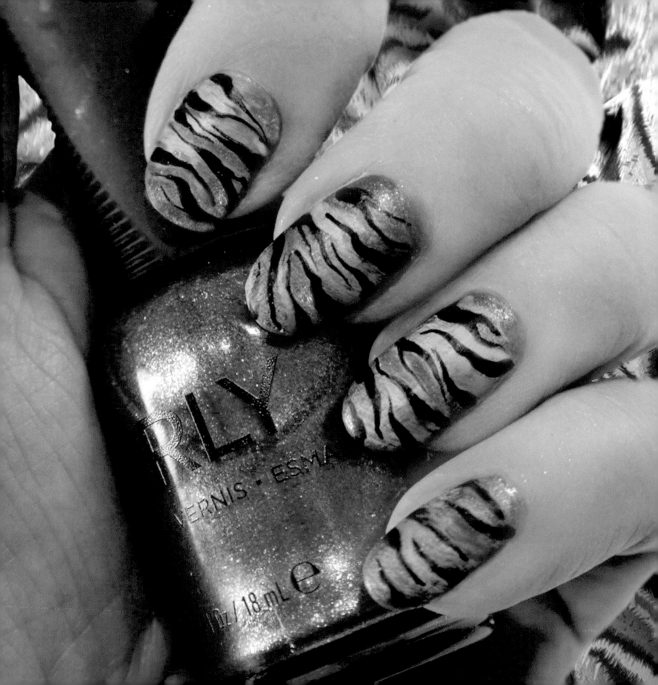

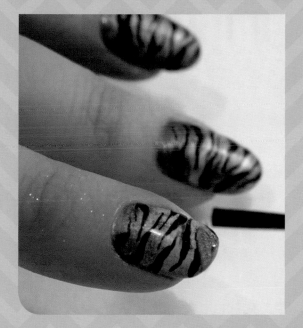

Top tip

For a funkier style, create the tiger stripes on the ring fingernails only, then use the shades in the project on each of the other nails to produce random designs.

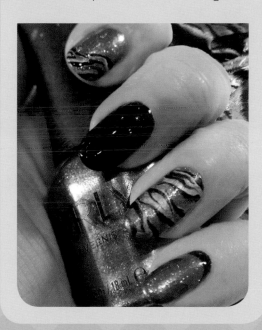

5 Apply a matte top coat to all nails for a softer, more realistic finish.

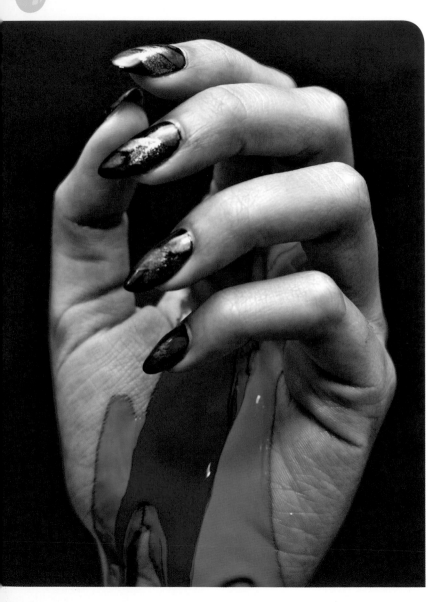

Image gallery

Left A colourful design on almond-shaped nails, inspired by dripping paint, by Ami Vega.

Below Ombré effect nails with striking white freehand nail art effects, by Ami Vega.

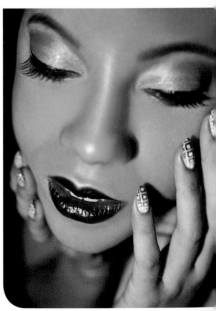

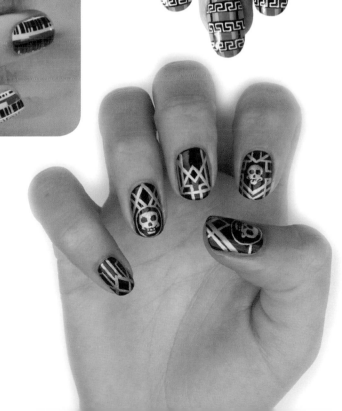

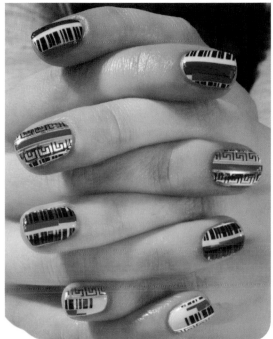

Above Minx nails in the colourful Barcode Maze design, applied by Leah Light.

Above right A colourful, stripy nail design with a hand-painted black-and-white Greek style overlay, by Sophie Harris-Greenslade.

Right Nails painted in black and adorned with a design inspired by Gothic architecture, by Sophie Harris-Greenslade.

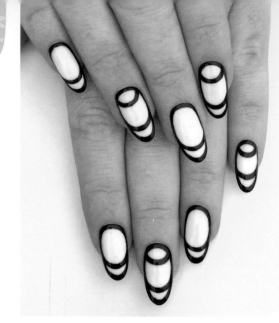

Left A combination of monochrome designs for a random, eye-catching nail effect, by Sophie Harris-Greenslade.

Below left Art-inspired nails with a colourful brushstroke effect, by Sophie Harris-Greenslade.

Right Short blue, pink and green nails with blue glitter tips and effects, by Myrdith Leon-McCormack for *Teen Vogue*.

Below 'Heartbreaker' nails – nude with a red heart shape at the tip – designed by Henry Holland for Elegant Touch.

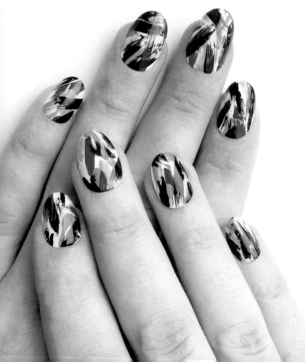

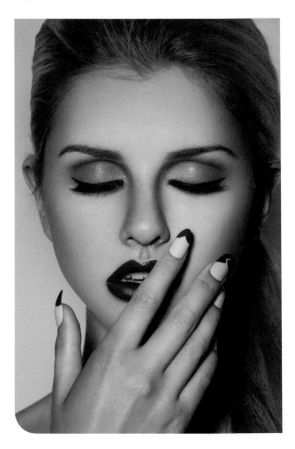

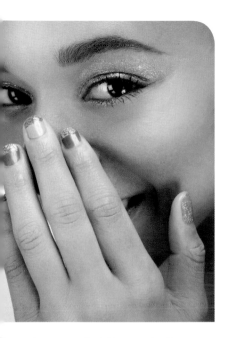

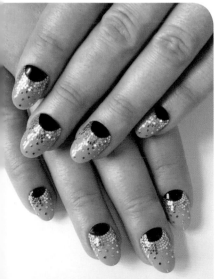

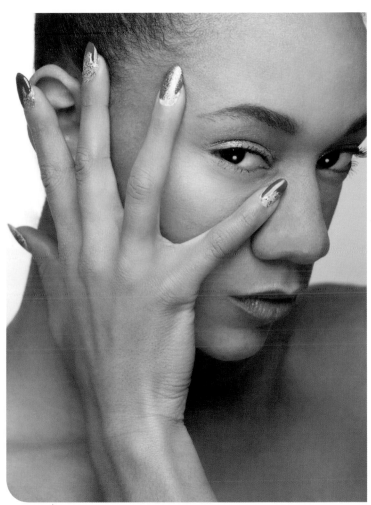

Left An elegant half moon nail design with gold embellishments. Created by Sophie Harris-Greenslade on nails shaped to the feminine almond.

Above Squoval nails with glitter effects, by Myrdith Leon-McCormack for *Teen Vogue*.

PROJECT:
HAWAIIAN FLORALS
by Sophie Harris-Greenslade

Create floral nails with bright colours on a dark base that are fun to wear all year round. Sophie Harris-Greenslade draws inspiration from Hawaiian flora for an eye-catching look.

You will need

- Base coat
- Black nail polish
- Nail art stripers or a thin artist's brush
- Nail art pens or nail polishes in fuchsia pink, yellow, light green, light blue, light pink, orange, black, white and dark green
- Dotting tool
- Top coat

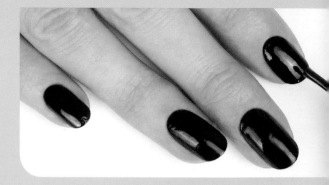

1 Apply the base coat, followed by two coats of black polish on all ten nails.

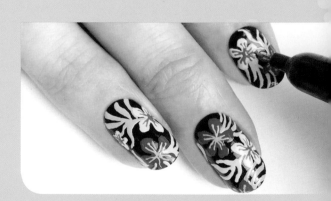

4 Using a light-pink nail art pen, paint detailing onto the fuchsia pink flowers. Repeat on the yellow flowers using an orange nail art pen.

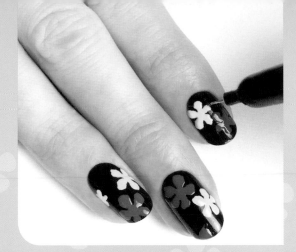

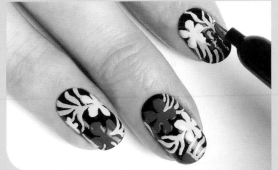

2 Using a fuchsia pink nail art pen or nail art brush dipped in fuchsia nail polish, paint five flowers randomly across the nails. When finished, repeat with the yellow polish.

3 Use a light-green nail art pen to paint tropical leaf shapes in between the flowers. Repeat in the remaining spaces with a light-blue nail art pen.

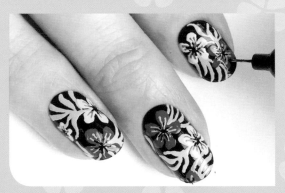

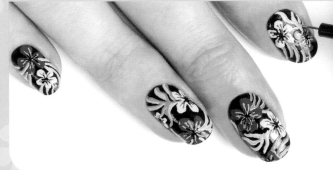

5 On top of the flower detailing, add little lines of black in the centre of the flowers using a black nail art pen.

6 Using a dark-green nail art pen, add shadow detailing to the green leaves. Do the same on the blue leaves using a light-green nail art pen.

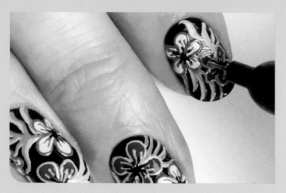
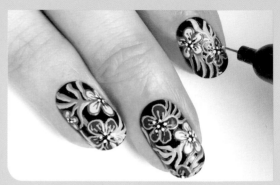

7 Outline the fuchsia flowers using a light-pink nail art pen, and outline the yellow flowers using an orange nail art pen.

8 Use a white nail art pen or dotting tool dipped in white nail polish to add dot detailing to the centre of the flowers, on top of the black line detailing.

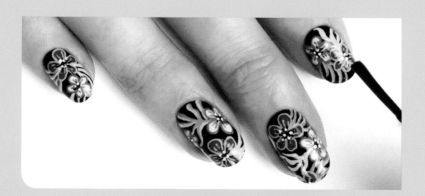

9 When the nails are dry, seal the design with a glossy top coat.

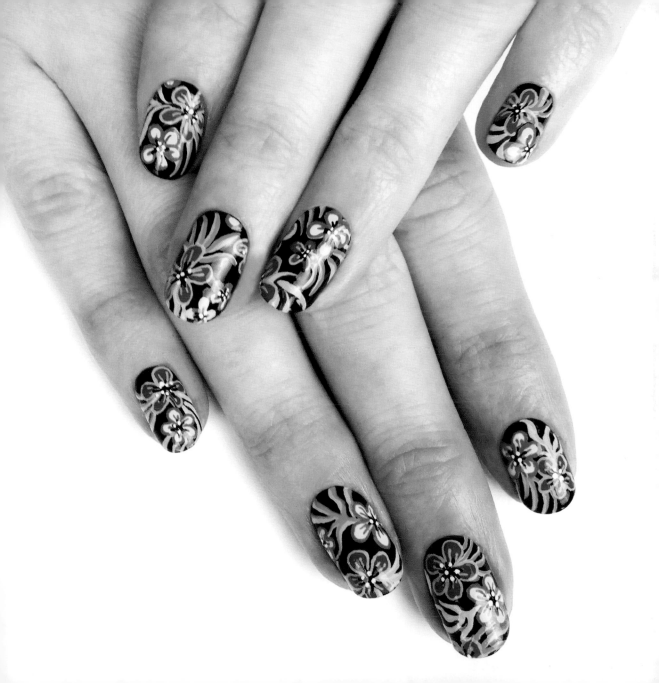

PROJECT: KALEIDOSCOPIC NAILS
by Sophie Harris-Greenslade

Complement an abundance of colour with an intricate design to really draw attention to nails. For this project, choose bright shades and a touch of sparkle to create an interesting, swirling design.

You will need

- Base coat
- White nail polish
- Nail art pens in pale pink, neon pink, silver glitter, blue, green, yellow and orange (or you can use nail polish and a thin brush)
- Top coat

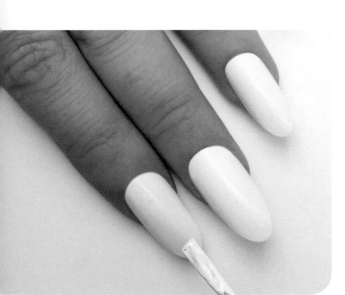

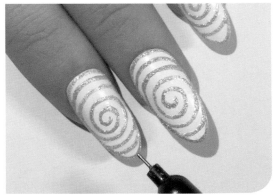

1 After applying a base coat, paint two coats of white nail polish on all nails.

2 Using a silver glitter nail art pen (or a brush dipped in silver glitter polish), draw a swirl from the middle of each nail all the way out to the edge. Draw an outline all the way round each nail.

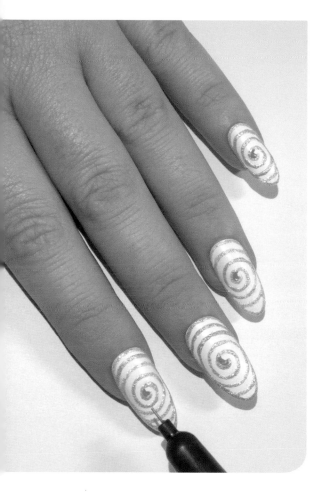

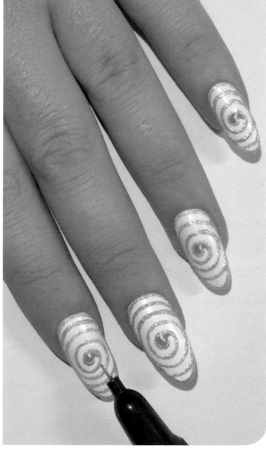

3 With a neon-pink nail art pen, draw a small crescent moon shape at the beginning of the swirl in the middle of the nail.

4 Leaving a small line of white, paint on another section using a green nail art pen. Each colour section needs to curve around the swirl in a crescent shape.

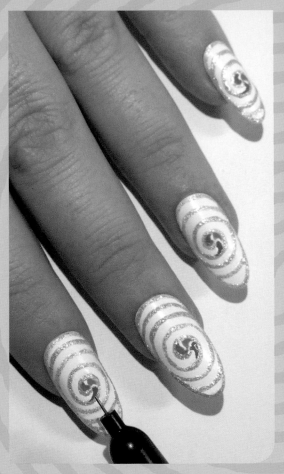

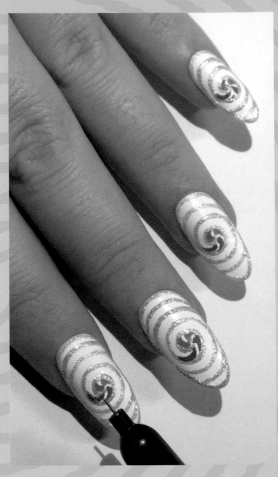

5 Leaving a small line of white, paint on a blue crescent section.

6 Repeat with orange, leaving a small line of white in between.

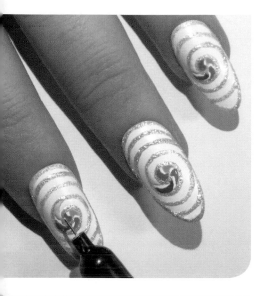

7 Repeat with yellow, following the silver glitter outline.

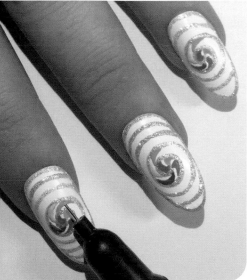

8 Continue to follow the outline on each nail and use a pale pink pen to create the next curved shape.

Top tips

- Practise designs with a nail art pen on paper before you start work on the nail

- Stay calm and relaxed throughout

- Steady your working arm on an armrest or with your other arm

- Seek inspiration everywhere, from television to fashion and nature

- Black and white polishes are great as a canvas – keep two of each in case one bottle runs out or is broken

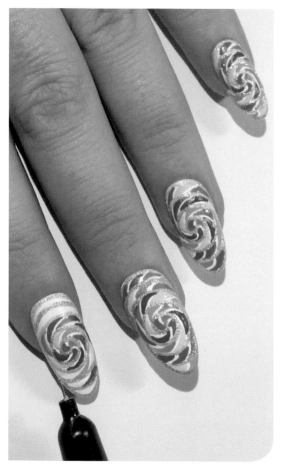

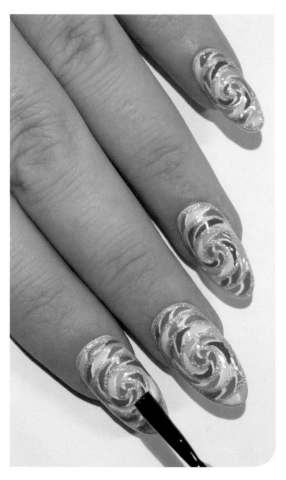

9 Repeat all the way round the swirl until you have filled the whole nail. You can use different colours if you like.

10 Finish the nails by applying a top coat.

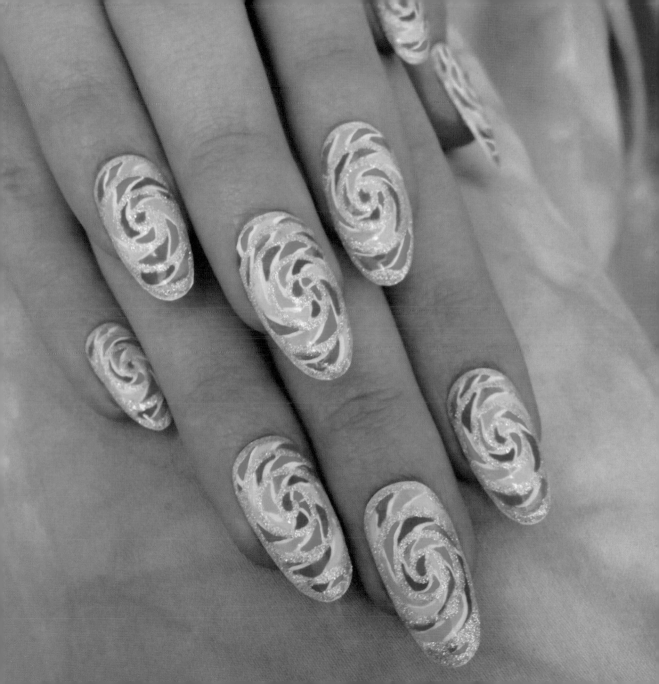

PROJECT: METALLIC CROSS NAILS
by Sophie Harris-Greenslade

Blood red and deep violet shades of polish, together with Gothic styles of architecture and art, such as pointed arches, crosses and carvings, can be used to great effect in nail design. This project demonstrates how to translate these dark shades and cross shapes onto nails.

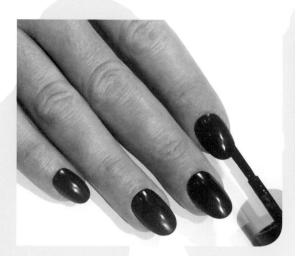

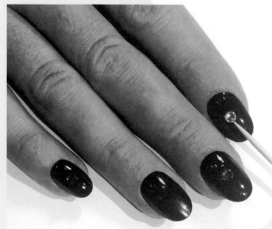

1 Apply a base coat and two thin coats of black nail polish to the nails.

2 Place a small dot of top coat in the centre of all the nails apart from the ring fingers. Use a cocktail stick to place a coloured gem on each dot of top coat and press down to secure.

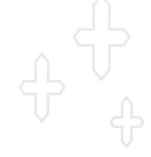

You will need

- Base coat
- Black nail polish
- Top coat
- Cocktail stick
- Coloured gems or crystals
- Scissors
- Gold metallic striping tape
- Small silver bullion beads
- Gold metallic flat stones
- Bronze striping tape

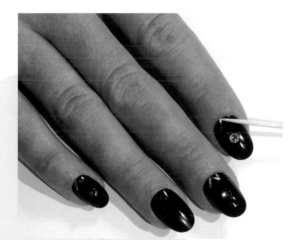

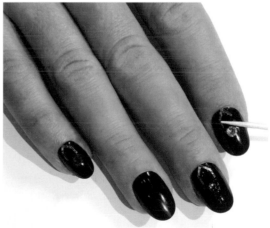

3 Cut two small strips of gold metallic striping tape. Use the top coat and a cocktail stick to place the tape in an upside-down V-shape in the centre of the base of the nail. Repeat on every nail that features a gem.

4 Cut two more small strips of striping tape and place vertically on the ends of the V-shape.

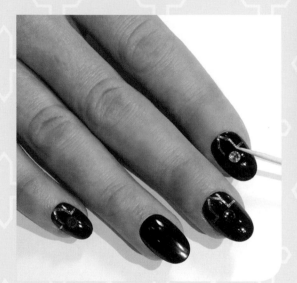

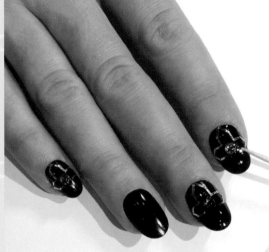

5 Cut two more small strips of gold tape and place horizontally at the ends of the vertical strips.

6 Place V-shapes of gold tape at either side of each gem. Add two more horizontal strips at the ends of the V-shapes to form the arms of the cross.

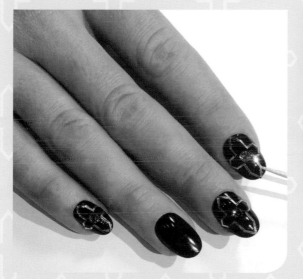

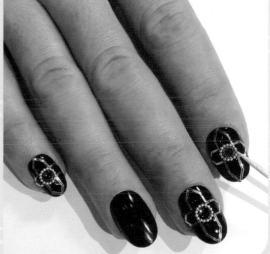

7 Add vertical strips of tape and a V-shape at the tip of the nail to finish off the cross shape.

8 Apply a layer of top coat to the eight nails with the cross design. Before it dries, add small silver bullion beads around each gem.

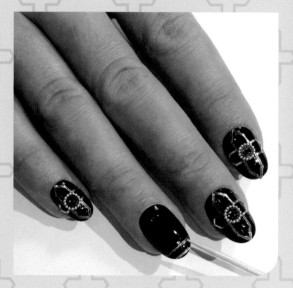

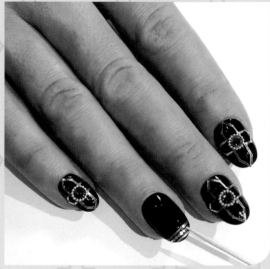

9 Apply top coat to the ring fingernails. Cut two strips of gold tape and place them horizontally at the tip of the nail, leaving a small gap in between.

10 In the gap between the tape, add flat gold metallic stones in a line across the nail.

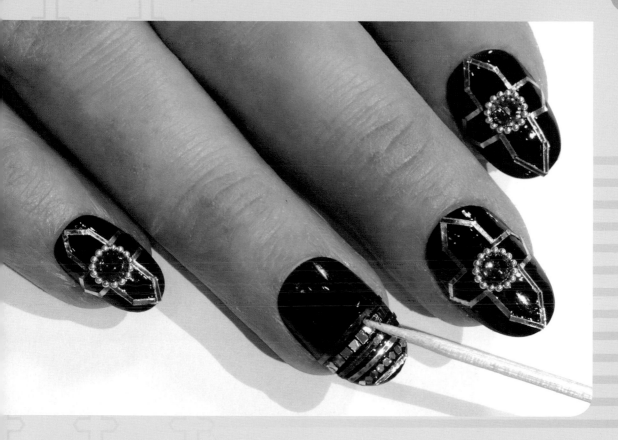

11 Cut two strips of bronze striping tape and place across the nail above the gold tape, leaving a gap in between. Cut small squares from the gold tape and place in the gap in a line, like a mosaic.

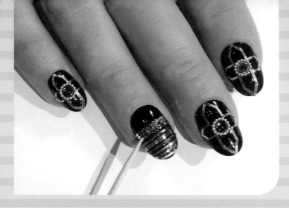

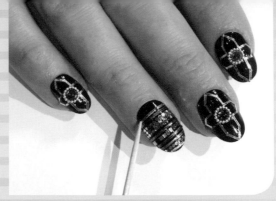

12 Add another layer of top coat, then place gold metallic flat stones in three lines above the bronze tape.

13 Above the lines of stones, add a bronze strip, followed by a gold one.

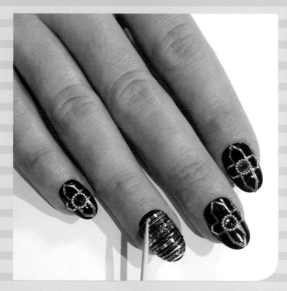

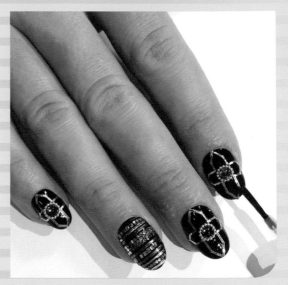

14 Cut the gold striping tape to short equal-sized lengths, creating small gold squares. Place these in a line across the nail above the bronze and gold strips.

15 Apply a final layer of top coat to all the nails.

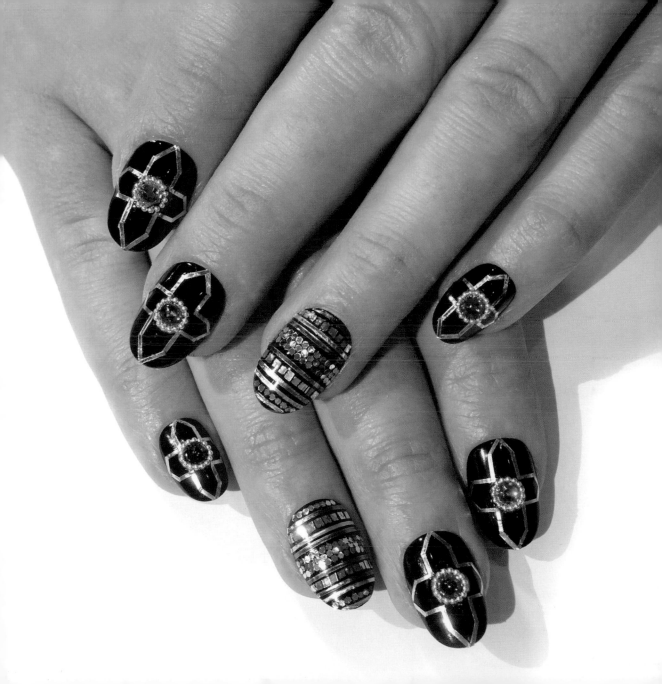

Picture credits

half title, Helena Biggs; *facing title*, Sophie Harris-Greenslade; *imprint*, Sophie Harris-Greenslade; *contents*, Sophie Harris-Greenslade; 6 Eva Darabos; 7 Sam Biddle; 8 Sam Biddle; 9 Shutterstock; 10 Shutterstock; 14 Shutterstock; 15 Nubar UK; 16–17 (*left to right*) Kimmie Kyees, Christina Rinaldi, Ami Vega; 22–3 Supa Nails; 26–7 Gerrard International/Jessica UK; 28–9 Leighton Denny Expert Nails; 30–31 (*clockwise from left*) Shutterstock, Bio Sculpture Gel UK, Ami Vega, Bio Sculpture Gel UK, Christina Rinaldi; 32–3 Leah Light; 34 (*clockwise from left*) Fleury Rose, Sam Biddle, Fleury Rose; 35 Leah Light; 36–7 Sam Biddle; 38 (*clockwise from left*) Sophie Harris-Greenslade x 2, Megumi Mizuno; 39 (*clockwise from top*) Leah Light x 2, Gemma Lambert; 40–43 Lena White Ltd/OPI UK; 44 (*clockwise from top left*) Leah Light, Ami Vega, Leah Light; 45 (*clockwise from top left*) Leah Light, Sophie Harris-Greenslade, Ami Vega, Christina Rinaldi; 46–7 Gemma Lambert; 48–51 Samantha Morales; 52–5 Helena Biggs; 56 (*left*) Ami Vega, (*right*) Fleury Rose; 57 Sophie Harris-Greenslade, Ami Vega, Christina Rinaldi; 58–61 Emil Baez; 62–3 Christina Rinaldi; 64 all Christina Rinaldi, apart from *top left* © Samantha Morales; 65 all Christina Rinaldi apart from *top left* © Sophie Harris-Greenslade; 66–9 Fleury Rose; 70 (*clockwise from left*) Charlotte Green, Sophie Harris-Greenslade x 2; 71 Sophie Harris-Greenslade; 72–3 Rock Cosmetics/Nail Rock; 74 (*clockwise from left*) Becky Maynes, Rock Cosmetics/Nail Rock x 2; 75 (*clockwise from top left*) www.vitaljuice.com, Naja Rickette, Rock Cosmetics/Nail Rock, Brandon Showers; 76–85 Sam Biddle; 86–9 Denise Wright; 90 (*clockwise from top left*) Ciaté, Sam Biddle, Sophie Harris-Greenslade, Ami Vega; 91 (*clockwise from top left*) Sophie Harris-Greenslade, Sam Biddle, Sophie Harris-Greenslade, Eva Darabos; 92–5 Eva Darabos; 96–9 Charlotte Green; 100 (*clockwise from left*) Samatha Morales, Fleury Rose, Sophie Harris-Greenslade; 101 (*clockwise from top left*) Samantha Morales, Sophie Harris-Greenslade, Samantha Morales; 102–105 Sam Biddle; 106 Samantha Morales; 107 (*clockwise from left*) Leah Light, Sophie Harris-Greenslade x 2; 108 (*clockwise from top left*) Sophie Harris-Greenslade, House of Holland for Elegant Touch, Sophie Harris-Greenslade; 109 (*clockwise from top left*) Vital Agibalow for *Teen Vogue* x 2, Sophie Harris-Greenslade; 110–127 Sophie Harris-Greenslade.

Stockists

Art Club/Color Club www.cosmeticgroup.com

Be Creative www.sambiddle.co.uk

Bio Sculpture Gel UK www.biosculpture.co.uk

China Glaze www.chinaglaze.com / www.thebeautypartnership.co.uk

Chronicle Stones www.chroniclestones.com

Ciaté www.ciate.co.uk

CND www.cnd.com / www.sweetsquared.com

Cult Nails www.cultnails.com

Elegant Touch www.eleganttouch.co.uk

Essie www.essie.com / www.essie.co.uk

Leighton Denny Expert Nails www.leightondennyexpertnails.com

Lumos/Famous Names www.famousnamesproducts.com / www.sweetsquared.com

Minx www.minxnails.com

Nail Rock www.rockbeautylondon.com

Nazila Love Glamour www.nazilaloveglamour.com

Nubar www.palmsextra.com

OPI www.opi.com / www.opiuk.com

Orly www.orlybeauty.com / www.graftonsbeauty.co.uk

Seche www.seche.com / www.louellabelle.co.uk

Supa Nails www.supanails.tumblr.com

Toma www.madbeauty.com